WHOLE FOOD BABY FOOD

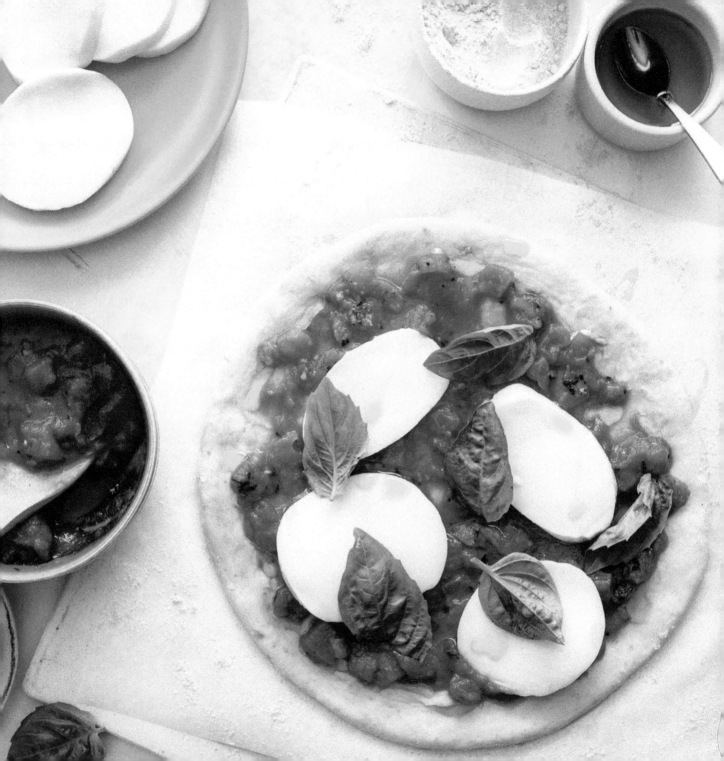

Whole Food Baby Food

Healthy Recipes to Help Infants and Toddlers Thrive

Laura Morton, MS, RDN, LD,
and Ellen Gipson, MA, RDN, LD

Photography by Annie Martin

ROCKRIDGE
PRESS

For general information on our other products and services or to obtain technical support, please contact our Customer Care Department within the United States at (866) 744-2665, or outside the United States at (510) 253-0500.

Rockridge Press publishes its books in a variety of electronic and print formats. Some content that appears in print may not be available in electronic books, and vice versa.

Interior and Cover Designer: Scott Petrower
Art Producer: Janice Ackerman
Editor: Kayla Park
Production Manager: Martin Worthington
Production Editor: Sigi Nacson

Photography: © 2020 Annie Martin
Food Styling by Oscar Molinar
Author Photo Laura Morton: © 2020 Ruthie Wolf
Author Photo Ellen Gipson: © 2020 Kendra Jane Photography

ISBN: Print 978-1-64739-858-3 | Ebook 978-1-64739-859-0
R0

To our adventurous eaters

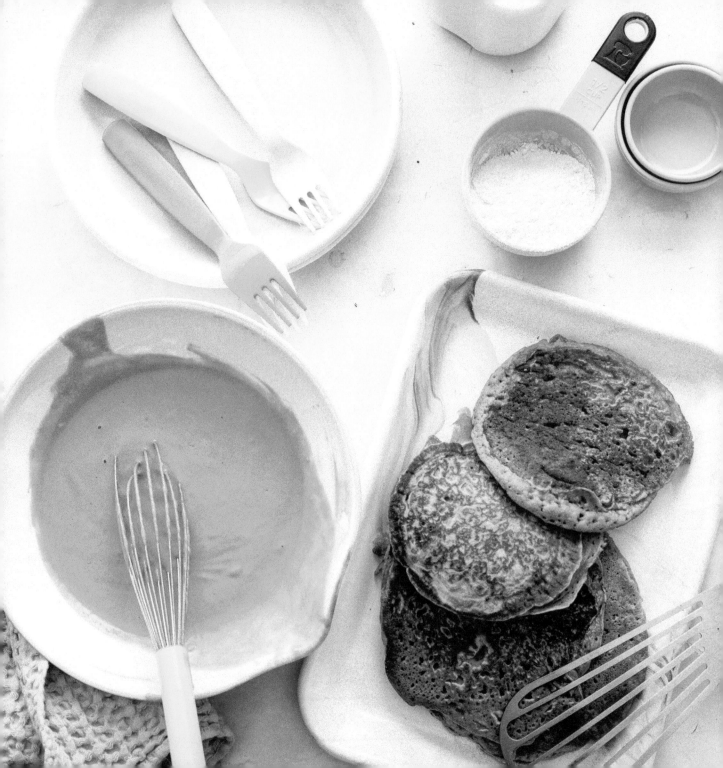

Contents

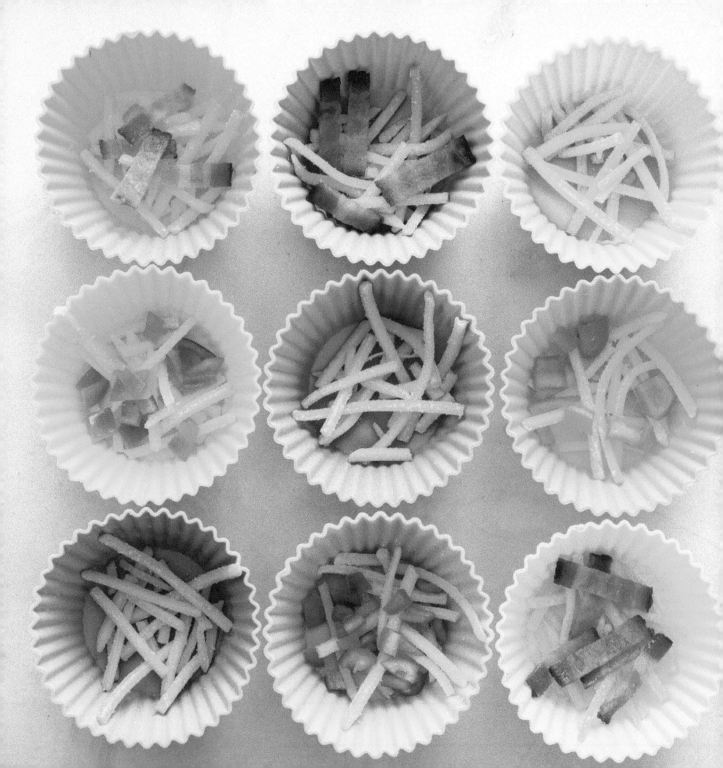

Introduction

Welcome to *Whole Food Baby Food*! We're thrilled that you're here to learn about something so important to us and our families: encouraging our little ones to love eating nourishing whole foods right from the start. Both of our babies got their start with whole foods like butternut squash, tender cooked beef, and even buttery corn on the cob! This all might sound great, but as registered dietitians working with little ones, we know the question on many parents' minds is "How do I even get started?"

The truth is there isn't one definitive approach to introducing solids, because all babies and families are unique. Furthermore, since baby food was invented about a century ago, methods of introduction have changed dramatically, and we can be pretty certain they will continue to change in the future. But there is one element that is likely to stay the same: whole, real, nourishing foods will always be the best bet. By beginning with whole foods and following your baby's cues, you'll have more control over the quality, nutrients, and flavors your little one is first exposed to.

This book will help you begin that wacky, messy, exciting journey into solids using a flexible approach that focuses on nutrient-dense whole foods introduced in the way that feels best for your family. It will guide you through everything you need to know about following baby's cues, food allergies, and making sure baby is getting all of the necessary nutrients. We begin with recipes for purees that focus on key nutrients for babies. Then we move on to combination and chunky purees, and we've got you covered with plenty of tried-and-true recipes for staple meals and snacks that we know you'll use long after your sweet baby's first birthday.

We're so excited that your family chose to introduce solids the whole food way. Welcome to the table, baby!

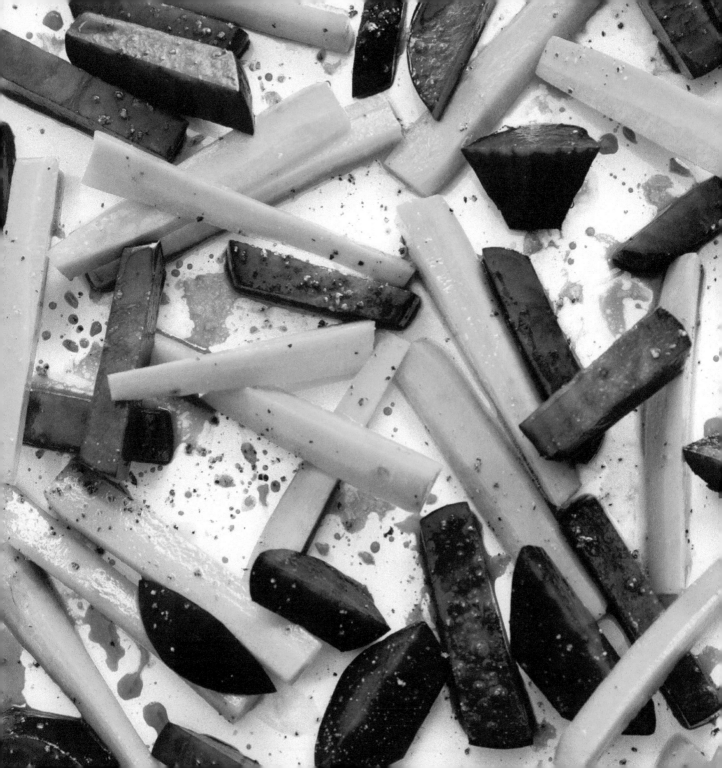

CHAPTER 1

Whole Foods Are the Best Foods

Introducing solid foods is an exciting and unique milestone—exciting because food is involved (and we *love* food), and unique because parents play such an important role. There is a lot of information available on what is the "best" way to introduce your baby to the wonderful world of food, but in reality, the best one is what works for your family. In this chapter, we will provide you with the need-to-know information, like why nutrient-packed whole foods are so important, what to look for when you're shopping (and what to avoid), how to determine portion sizes, how to deal with picky eaters, and what the latest research tells us on allergy prevention—all so that you can confidently and joyfully welcome your little one to the table.

WHAT ARE WHOLE FOODS?

What exactly do we mean by whole foods? Although the definition is flexible, for us, whole foods are foods that are as close as possible to how you might find them in nature. Cooking with whole foods means going back to basics and introducing real, minimally processed whole foods right from the start.

That said, our definition definitely doesn't have to be all or nothing. Cooking with whole foods can mean ditching heavily processed packaged food as often as possible, while still loving the convenience of creamy store-bought yogurt and picked-at-their-peak frozen peas. We believe a flexible and inclusive approach to eating is important, especially when little eyes are watching. Our goal is to lay the groundwork so you can decide for your own family just what whole foods mean to you.

WHOLE FOODS: EVERYONE BENEFITS

Many babies get their start with mostly whole foods. It usually isn't until a little later that the processed foods, cleverly advertised as baby-friendly, sneak in. There are numerous reasons to aim for a lifestyle rich in whole foods, including the following:

Nutrient density: Foods in their whole form provide a range of beneficial nutrients and other components, like enzymes and fiber, designed to work together. There are several nutrients found in whole foods that are especially important for babies, which we highlight in "Nutrition at Every Stage" (page 12) and in the recipe headnotes.

Flavor exposure: When offering your baby whole foods, the focus is on bringing out the flavor of the actual food (even if that food is bitter—we're looking at you, broccoli). Many prepackaged baby foods mask bitter vegetables by combining them with sweet fruit flavors. Learning to accept bitter flavors is an important part of early exposure and will set up baby to enjoy complex tastes later in life.

Variety: The exposure to a variety of flavors during a short period of time in baby's early life may decrease the likelihood of picky eating in later stages. The result is a little one who is more likely to accept a variety of foods as they grow and a family that is expanding their whole food experience together.

Healthy relationship with food: One of the most important parts of introducing solids, no matter what food you begin with, is allowing a healthy relationship with food to grow. Responsive feeding (see page 13), early flavor and texture exposure, and a positive family food culture set the stage for a lifelong healthy relationship with food.

No additives: Choosing whole foods is a great way to automatically avoid added sugar and salt in baby's diet. Limiting the introduction of processed foods also helps avoid additives and synthetic ingredients such as artificial sweeteners, colors, flavors, and preservatives.

CHOOSING AND SHOPPING

Contrary to what we often hear, whole foods prepared at home can be much less expensive, and at the same time much higher quality, than prepackaged versions of common infant and toddler foods. Take these comparisons, for example:

	WHOLE FOOD DATE-BASED GRANOLA BARS (10 BARS)	1 (12-INCH) MARGHERITA PIZZA	1 (6-OUNCE) VEGETARIAN BEAN BURRITO	TEETHING BISCUITS (24 BISCUITS)
Homemade	$2.89	$1.74	$0.57	$1.27
Store-bought/ prepackaged	$9.89	$6.19	$2.99	$4.64

Store-bought prices from the Target app, May 2020. Homemade prices based on ingredient cost and weight; ingredients purchased from Target, May 2020.

Although a whole food diet does mean spending a bit more time in the kitchen, the recipes in this book are designed to come together quickly. And, by cooking at home, you're imparting an understanding of where foods come from and how they are prepared, which is a huge benefit for little ones.

What to Look For

When you are selecting whole foods for your family, you may be wondering if you should always choose organic or non-GMO, and what these labels actually mean. These topics are hotly debated and for good reason: they are complex and involve something very personal, our food. The bottom line is choosing whole foods, especially fruits and vegetables, that will supply your baby and your family with the nutrients they need, while minimizing the additives they don't.

ORGANIC

Not all whole foods are organic, and all organic foods are not necessarily whole. Organic refers to the way a plant or animal was grown or raised, but there are organic products that are highly processed, like snack foods, candy, and sugary cereals. Although whole food is food that has been minimally processed, it doesn't necessarily mean it was grown or raised according to organic standards.

Organic plant foods are grown without most synthetic pesticides and fertilizers, growth hormones, irradiation, and genetic engineering. Organic certification for meat, poultry, dairy, and fish signifies that the animals have been raised in living conditions close to how they would naturally live, fed 100 percent organic feed, and never given antibiotics or growth hormones. Following these practices is more expensive, as is receiving the US Department of Agriculture (USDA) Organic seal, which is why organic foods are generally more costly.

An alternative to seeking out organic labels in the grocery store is purchasing whole food locally, through farmers' markets, community-supported agriculture (CSA), and directly from local farmers. This is often more affordable and environmentally friendly than purchasing organic foods at the supermarket, and it can even provide more nutrient-dense foods.

Whether you decide on organic, conventional, or a combination is completely up to you. Even as nutrition pros, we have differing preferences, but both of us prioritize a variety of nutrient-packed whole foods to fuel our families.

NON-GMO AND OTHER ACRONYMS

Genetically modified organism (GMO) is a catchall term for many different types of genetic engineering, but as it pertains to food, it is basically a plant or animal whose DNA has been modified in order to improve an outcome—for example, to increase yield or disease resistance.

Because GMOs have been in the food supply only since 1994, many people are concerned about the lack of long-term data on potential health effects of GMO consumption. On the other hand, many major organizations, including the World Health Organization (WHO), agree that there is a lack of evidence to date for potential adverse health effects and recognize GMOs as safe to consume.

Foods containing GMOs currently do not require a label in the United States, though many companies use a "non-GMO" label to assure concerned consumers there are no genetically modified ingredients in their products and perhaps to gain a competitive edge.

If your family chooses to avoid genetically modified foods, it can be done by choosing foods with a USDA Organic label, or even better, getting to know the local growers in your area and finding out firsthand how their products are grown.

HORMONES AND ANTIBIOTICS

Though naturally occurring hormones are present in different quantities in both plant and animal foods, added hormones, including estrogen, testosterone, and their synthetic versions, have been approved for use in cattle and sheep since the 1950s with the goal of faster and more efficient animal growth. According to the USDA, added hormones are not used in the production of poultry or pork. Hormones are rarely given to dairy cattle in the United States today, due to consumer backlash over the use of an added hormone called rBST, which was used to increase milk supply.

Because naturally occurring hormones are present in all of these animal foods, as well as in many plant foods, a "hormone-free" label doesn't hold a lot of meaning. Similar to GMOs, there is debate over the safety of added synthetic or natural hormones in the food supply; however, consensus from large organizations such as the Food and Drug Administration (FDA) assures the public of the safety of the practice.

According to the Centers for Disease Control and Prevention (CDC), the use of antibiotics for growth promotion has been banned in the United States, so no animals should be receiving antibiotics unless they need it to treat an infection, and if antibiotics must be administered, levels are strictly monitored, and all meat should be antibiotic-free by the time it reaches the grocery store—whether or not there is an "antibiotic-free" label on it. Organically raised animals are never given antibiotics or hormones, so families wishing to avoid these altogether can choose organic.

MARKETING BUZZWORDS

Whole foods don't have many health claims on the label when compared with highly processed foods—and this is a good thing. Often, the more health claims the product has, the more unhealthy attributes it may be trying to cover up.

Some claims that appear on food labels are regulated ("excellent source of vitamin C," "USDA Organic," "no added salt"), whereas others can be misleading ("natural," "made with real fruit," "farm raised").

For a more truthful glimpse into the health benefits of a packaged food, check out the ingredients list. Is sugar or one of its synonyms (including brown rice syrup, high fructose corn syrup, malt syrup, and anything ending in "-ose") at the top of the list? Are there hydrogenated oils? Unfamiliar preservatives? When shopping for whole foods, look for a short list of easy-to-recognize ingredients and no added sugar.

Specific Foods

Not all food processing is a bad thing. Some, like pasteurization, are major factors in ensuring the safety of our food supply. Below is a list of minimally processed staples, many of which you will see in the recipes in this book:

- Bread (look for a short ingredients list)
- Butter, unsalted
- Canned (low sodium) and dried beans*
- Canned oysters, salmon, sardines, tuna*
- Canned tomato products (no sodium added), like diced tomatoes and tomato paste*
- Cooking oil (coconut, olive, avocado, etc.)
- Dried herbs and spices
- Frozen fruits and vegetables
- Meat and fish
- Nuts, seeds, and nut butters
- Pasta
- Unsweetened dried fruit
- Whole-grain and unbleached all-purpose flour
- Whole grains like quinoa and old-fashioned rolled or quick-cooking oats
- Whole milk yogurt, cheese, and milk

*When choosing canned foods, we do pay attention to one label claim: BPA-free liner. This may appear on the label or printed on top of the can.

FAMILY FOOD CULTURE

One of the most important long-term goals with feeding baby is raising them to have a positive and robust relationship with food. Building a strong culture around whole foods at home can mean so many different things, but here are a few tangible ideas to get started:

Cook and eat meals together at home. This can mean using recipes that have been in your family for generations and/or starting from scratch with your own collection of favorites.

Involve kids in cooking from an early age. Granted it can be messy, but even babies as young as one can play a role. The result is children who grow up comfortable in the kitchen and understand the part food plays in fueling our families. They may even end up with a passion for cooking.

Make home a safe haven from excessive food marketing exposure. Familiarize kids with whole foods from an early age. This involves a balance of teaching kids that certain foods (like packaged, highly processed foods or fast food) are not beneficial for their growing bodies, without demonizing or completely banning these foods; the role of these foods in our lives can be simply for enjoyment from time to time.

Food = Fun

Let's refocus on what really matters here. Finding the joy in food. All foods. Whole foods. As a caregiver, your main role is to create a safe, supportive feeding environment that fosters an exploration and discovery of food. Focusing on whole foods opens baby to endless flavor combinations, vibrant colors, intriguing textures, and health-sustaining nutrients. This is a fundamental milestone in baby's development, a skill set they will use the rest of their lives, and, best of all, you get to be a part of it.

PUREES AND BABY-LED WEANING/FEEDING

Even just 10 years ago, the recommended age to begin solids was around 4 months (and before that, even earlier!), thus purees were the only possible way to begin. However, now all major health organizations, including the American Academy of Pediatrics (AAP), the Academy of Nutrition and Dietetics, and the WHO, agree that the optimal age to introduce solids is 6 months; before then, they support the use of breast milk and/or formula exclusively.

Families are now choosing more whole, natural, simple unprocessed foods, and many are learning to make their own pureed baby foods from whole foods, like the recipes in this book, or are reaching back into a very old but recently revolutionized feeding philosophy called baby-led weaning (BLW). Regardless of whether you start with purees or BLW, we encourage you to prioritize family mealtimes, strive to follow responsive feeding cues, understand the parents' versus child's role at mealtimes, and, most important, create an environment that fosters a healthy relationship with food. For many, beginning with purees can help ensure baby is actually consuming the nutrients offered and is a way to ease parents' fears of baby choking. For others, the convenience of BLW makes it an obvious fit. Following are brief summaries of each approach to guide you in deciding which method is the best for your family.

Purees

The most common approach to starting solids is through the introduction of purees. The thin, smooth texture makes a seamless transition into baby's current diet of breast milk or formula. When baby is nearing the 6-month mark and has met the signs of readiness for solids (see "When Is Baby Ready?" opposite), it's time to get excited. At this point, you will be in a great position to begin responsive feeding (see page 13). The beginner puree recipes in this book focus on nutrient density and flavor exploration. We recommend keeping portions small (1 to 2 tablespoons) and focusing on identifying baby's satiety cues during mealtimes.

We encourage families not to offer *only* pureed textures for too long and suggest that families with healthy, full-term babies foster their child's instinctual adventurous eating by including purees alongside other textures within a few weeks of beginning solids at 6 months.

Baby-Led Weaning

In our first cookbook, *BLW Baby Food Cookbook*, we defined baby-led weaning as "the introduction of nutritious whole foods when baby shows interest and signs of readiness to self-feed." Like with traditional purees, complementary foods are introduced around 6 months of age, when baby is meeting the physical and mental developmental signs of readiness (see opposite). There aren't really special meals just for baby; instead, BLW typically begins with soft solids from the family table, then infants rely on their self-feeding skills and intuition to regulate the amount of food needed to grow. We like to think of BLW as an approach to feeding without the strict guidelines of stages and progressions. Baby leads through textural transitions. Think of BLW as a back-to-basics approach to mealtimes, before the influence of a commercial baby food industry.

WHEN IS BABY READY?

Do you know who is the absolute best source for determining if baby is ready for solids? Baby! As baby nears 6 months of age, look for the following distinct signs indicating readiness for solid food. For the greatest success in responsive feeding, baby should be exhibiting most or all of these indicators.

Sitting up. Baby can sit with little or no support. Stability of major muscle groups will foster a safe swallow.

Head control. Baby can maintain good head and neck control while sitting in a high chair.

Hand control. Fine motor skills are developing when infants can see and pick up an item with intention. This is typically followed by bringing items to the mouth for chewing or teething.

Diminished tongue thrust. Spitting or pushing food out of the mouth is commonly misidentified as meaning dislike for a particular food. But infants are born with a protective reflex that triggers the tongue to thrust forward at the weight of even the thinnest purees. This reflex typically diminishes around 6 months.

Interest in food and desire to eat. Typically, this is the last piece of the puzzle to develop. Look for a true interest in wanting something more, something with substance, something for their own—a natural appetite. They may open their mouth or lean forward when food is offered or try to grab the spoon from your hands. By this point, let them have at it!

Spices and Flavors

Did you know baby's food doesn't have to be bland? Beginning with flavorful foods establishes a norm of expectancy in baby, helping them grow into adventurous eaters. We want to stimulate their taste buds and expand their palate by incorporating a variety of flavors. Herbs and spices add color, fragrance, and flavor to our foods. There is a difference between hot and aromatic spices, and we'll include the latter along with herbs early on in baby's meal. These can be mixed into a variety of purees; sprinkled onto soft, chunky solids; infused into cooking oils; or marinated onto tender meats. Additional ideas for introducing baby to exciting flavor combinations can be found in the Healthy Meal Builder (page 145).

NUTRITION AT EVERY STAGE

After 6 months, the order in which foods are introduced isn't as important as keeping a focus on variety. The old recommendation called for waiting days between new food introduction to watch for potential allergic reactions, but there is no evidence that this waiting period poses any benefit. Pacing food introduction can also cause parents to miss out on a crucial window of flavor exposure.

For the first year, the majority of babies' nutritional needs are being met with breast milk or formula. Remembering this can take some of the pressure off while baby is taking their time getting the hang of eating solid foods. There are a few important nutrients to keep in mind when introducing solids: iron, zinc, fat, and vitamin D.* Including food sources of these specific nutrients every day is a straightforward way to meet nutritional goals, which is why the recipes in this book are designed with these nutrients in mind.

The AAP recommends all infants and children take a daily vitamin D supplement of at least 400 IU beginning shortly after birth.

Foods to Avoid in the First Year

We want parents to feel liberty and excitement in introducing solids, but this process should also be grounded in science to keep baby safe. Here is a short but important list of foods to avoid in the first year.

Cow's milk (to drink): While baby is under 1 year old, breast milk and/or formula should be their only source of fluid calories. The nutrient makeup of cow's milk can cause problems with nutrient and calorie absorption. Cow's milk can be used in recipes, however. Dairy products such as cheese and yogurt can be included from 6 months on. (See "Allergies and Sensitivities," page 15, for more information on how to safely start these foods.)

Fruit juice: The AAP recommends that no fruit juice be given to babies younger than a year old because there is no nutritional benefit, and it can lead to excessive weight gain and tooth decay.

Honey: Honey and foods including honey should be avoided until around 12 months, when a child's gut can handle the very small but serious risk of botulism spores in honey.

Salt: Consuming too much sodium can be a problem for adults and little ones alike. The CDC estimates more than 70 percent of excess sodium comes from processed foods, so introducing baby to whole foods without added salt is a good idea for keeping their salt intake low.

Portion Sizes and Feeding Styles

Understanding your role and baby's role at mealtimes is an essential component for success. Responsive feeding means trusting baby to regulate their own intake, even when they eat more or less than we think they need. The division of responsibility (a phrase coined by child nutrition expert Ellyn Satter) reminds parents that they are in charge of choosing what food is served and where it is eaten, and little ones are in charge of how much and even if they eat at any particular meal. Since calorie needs are being met through breast milk or formula, the amount of food consumed is not critical. During the first few weeks, keep portion sizes small (1 to 2 tablespoons) so as not to overwhelm them. Babies are great communicators and will let you know if they're hungry for more or if they're done. Watch for their cues, and keep mealtimes positive.

Babies may occasionally gag during mealtimes, but do not be alarmed. Infants' gag reflex is much more sensitive than that of adults. The gag is a safety mechanism that moves unchewed food back toward the front of the mouth so it can be re-chewed. Experiencing a new texture or flavor is a common trigger. If gagging occurs, remain calm and try not to interfere by picking up baby or taking food from the mouth. You can help by removing any food in front of baby, so they don't try to put more in, and allowing them to concentrate on the piece in their mouth. These episodes cause more stress for parents than baby.

Picky Eaters

Pickiness is a normal part of development and should be anticipated but not catered to. Most children are born with the ability to self-regulate their appetites based on the needs of their growing body. There are many pieces to this puzzle. External factors like physical environment (being in a new location), social environment (eating with friends), distractions (watching TV), mealtime engagement (eating alone versus with family), and meal timing (snacking too close to mealtime) can influence appetite, as can internal factors like sleep, hydration, cognitive development (toddler looking to express independence), or health (sickness, fevers, teething, painful bowel movements, breathing difficulty/congestion, etc.). Try not to interpret rejection of a particular food for dislike and stop offering it; instead, provide continual and regular exposure to a wide variety of foods.

ALLERGIES AND SENSITIVITIES

When parents begin introducing solids, we encourage them to avoid overanalyzing the what-ifs. Currently, about 5 percent of children 5 years and younger have a food allergy, and about 90 percent of all food allergies are caused by the following nine foods: milk, eggs, wheat, soy, tree nuts, peanuts, fish, shellfish, and, most recently, sesame. A food allergy happens when the body reacts, in ways ranging from mild to severe, to proteins found in foods. Many food allergies will be short term, and the child may grow out of them before puberty (especially in cases of egg, wheat, milk, and soy allergies).

It is no longer recommended to delay the introduction of potential allergens, but actually almost the opposite. Updated recommendations encourage early (around 6 months) and frequent introduction of allergens as a key to prevention. You can start with the beginner purees with no allergens included. Then, once baby has tolerated a few different foods, you're free to start with any of the potential allergens listed above. But, of course, check with your pediatrician first if you have any specific concerns about food allergies.

A unique frame of reference behind allergen introduction is to offer with intention. In this way you are careful, attentive, and observant during this process, conscious of the potential risk of activating an allergic response. We recommend intentional introduction using whole foods, so you are confident about the ingredients. Reactions typically happen within a short time after consumption, and key signs of potential allergic response include, but are not limited to, hives or eczema; sneezing; wheezing or difficulty breathing; swelling; nausea, vomiting, or diarrhea; light-headedness; and/or loss of consciousness.

Current guidelines consider babies with severe eczema, an egg allergy, or both to be at high risk for developing a peanut allergy. If this sounds familiar, check in with your pediatrician well before introducing solids; they may recommend introducing peanuts between 4 to 6 months. Older siblings with a peanut allergy may also increase the risk.

A WHOLE FOOD KITCHEN

Building a whole food kitchen doesn't have to happen overnight. But chances are you already have some delicious whole foods for baby in your kitchen.

To help you get started at the grocery store, we've put together this list of whole food kitchen staples, which you can customize based on your family's preferences. We have also included a list of equipment we use in our own kitchens that will come in handy for the recipes that follow. But rest assured, it is totally possible to get started without owning a lot of fancy gear.

Stocking the Pantry (and More)

Having a well-stocked pantry and fridge is the cornerstone of any whole food kitchen. The lists that follow include our go-to refrigerated, frozen, and pantry staples. These lists cover all the bases for first foods and for the recipes in this book.

When it comes to spices, we like to use a combination of fresh and dried, opting for spices from trustworthy brands when purchasing dried to reduce the likelihood of lead contamination, a common problem with imported herbs, especially those ordered from unfamiliar brands online.

CANNED GOODS

- Chunk white skipjack tuna, salmon, and oysters
- Crushed or diced tomatoes, no salt added
- Full-fat coconut milk

- Low-sodium beans, such as black beans, chickpeas, and white beans
- Low-sodium broth: chicken or vegetable
- Marinara sauce, no salt added

DRY GOODS

- Baking powder
- Baking soda
- Dried red, green, or brown lentils
- Old-fashioned rolled and quick-cooking oats
- Pasta, in a variety of shapes
- Quinoa
- Unbleached all-purpose flour
- Whole wheat flour

NUTS AND SEEDS

- Chia seeds
- Ground flaxseed
- Peanut, almond, sunflower, and/ or cashew butter and tahini (sesame seed paste)

OILS

- Avocado oil
- Extra-virgin olive oil
- Unrefined coconut oil

HERBS, SPICES, AND SEASONINGS

- Basil
- Black pepper
- Cilantro
- Cinnamon, ground
- Cumin, ground
- Dill
- Garlic powder
- Ginger, ground
- Oregano
- Parsley
- Rosemary
- Thyme
- Turmeric

PRODUCE

- Apples
- Avocados
- Bananas
- Beets
- Bell peppers (red or green)
- Berries
- Broccoli and cauliflower
- Carrots
- Fresh herbs
- Garlic
- Ginger
- Leafy greens
- Local seasonal produce
- Onions
- Potatoes
- Squash, including acorn, butternut, spaghetti squash, and zucchini
- Sweet potatoes

DAIRY PRODUCTS

- Butter
- Eggs
- Cheeses, including cheddar and Parmesan
- Plain whole milk yogurt
- Whole milk

MEAT, FISH, AND OTHER PROTEINS

- Chicken
- Beef
- Salmon
- Shrimp
- Tofu

FROZEN

- Bananas
- Berries
- Broccoli florets
- Carrots
- Cauliflower florets
- Corn
- Mangoes
- Peas
- Squash

Essential Tools and Equipment

Now that we've got the pantry and fridge stocked, let's talk tools and equipment. You can provide a diverse and delicious whole food experience for baby without all the hot new gadgets, something both of us know from our own experiences working in small kitchens. There are, however, a few things that may make it easier to get the job done. If you have a stocked kitchen already—woo-hoo! If not, don't sweat it. Feel free to get started anyway, and figure out what you need as you go.

PREP ·

- Blender or food processor: A good quality blender is great for baby food, and a food processor is often more powerful than a blender, if you have the space and budget for it.
- Box grater
- Dry measuring cups
- Fruit and vegetable peeler
- Glass liquid measuring cups
- Measuring spoons
- Set of nested mixing bowls: small, medium, and large (stainless steel works well to prevent chips or breaks)
- Sharp knife
- Silicone spatula
- Whisk
- Wooden spoons

- Baking pans: 9-by-13-inch and 8-by-8-inch (glass, ceramic, or stainless steel)
- Cast-iron skillet and Dutch oven: cast iron transfers dietary iron to whatever is cooked in it
- Mixer: handheld electric mixer or stand mixer
- Muffin tin
- Pie plate

- Rimmed baking sheets
- Saucepans: small, medium, and large (avoid nonstick surfaces)
- Skillets: small, medium, and large (avoid nonstick surfaces)
- Stockpot
- Unbleached parchment paper
- Waffle iron

- Glass jars with lids, including pint and quart sizes
- Glass or stainless-steel food-storage containers with tight-fitting lids

- Reusable zip-top bags
- Reusable plastic wrap or other food covering film
- Silicone or stainless-steel ice cube tray

ABOUT THE RECIPES

Ready to get cookin'? In the following chapters you will find recipes that take you from the first bite to baby's first birthday and beyond. We hope to inspire you with tasty flavor combinations in smooth and chunky textures as well as soft finger foods, all of which are great from 6 months on. We are big on family meals, so you'll find many recipes throughout the book that can be shared with everyone at the table.

Whether beginning with purees, finger foods, or a combination of both, the best outcomes result from feeding in a responsive way. Introducing solids almost always takes some figuring out to see what works best. Let baby take the lead and choose if they want to eat and how much at any given meal.

At the top of every recipe, you'll find a few handy labels that can help you make a quick decision about what to prepare. Whether you are interested in stocking the freezer, packing snacks for a road trip, or whipping up a nut-free snack to take to a playgroup, we've got you covered. In addition to dietary labels such as dairy-free, gluten-free, nut-free, vegan, and vegetarian, we have included the following:

Early Introduction: These recipes include one of the nine most common allergens.

Freezer-Friendly: These recipes freeze well.

Healthy Fats: There are plenty of healthy fats for baby in these recipes.

Iron-Rich: These recipes are a great source of iron.

No-Cook: Whip up these recipes without turning on the stove.

On the Go: These recipes are easy to pack up and take with you.

Quick and Easy: These recipes come together in 30 minutes or less.

Baby Guacamole, page 54

Creamy Tomato and
Chickpea Puree, page 46

Creamy Butternut Squash
with Rosemary, page 25

Spiced Pear Puree, page 28

Simple Salmon Puree, page 33

CHAPTER 2

Beginner Purees
(6 to 8 Months)

The recipes in this chapter are simple, nutrient-packed first purees for babies just getting started with solids. They were developed to emphasize flavor exposure, from earthy ingredients like broccoli, carrots, and lentils to savory proteins like salmon and liver.

Keep in mind that portion size varies from baby to baby. Begin with 1 to 2 tablespoons per meal, and follow baby's cues for more. At 6 months, you can begin with only purees or introduce chunky purees (chapter 3) and soft table foods (chapter 4) at the same time. Regardless of the texture of the first food, gagging is very common and usually subsides as your little one gets used to solids.

These recipes will typically make 1 to 2 cups of puree, though you may get a little more or less depending on the size of the fruits and vegetables that you use. To extend the life of your leftovers, you can spoon them into a silicone or stainless-steel ice cube tray and freeze until solid. Once frozen, transfer the cubes to a freezer-safe container or reusable zip-top bag. Before serving, remove a portion from the freezer and thaw it in the refrigerator overnight. Leftover cubes of frozen puree can also be stirred into soups and sauces or blended into a smoothie.

Creamy Butternut Squash with Rosemary

Butternut squash was a first food for each of our babies. It's naturally on the sweet side with a rich color—a clue that a fruit or vegetable is packed with nutrients. Well-cooked butternut squash can also be mashed with a fork or offered in strips from 6 months on.

1 (12-ounce) bag frozen cubed butternut squash

½ cup water, plus more as needed

2 tablespoons unsalted butter or coconut oil, melted

¼ teaspoon dried or chopped fresh rosemary

1. Preheat the oven to 375°F.
2. Put the squash on a rimmed baking sheet and bake for about 15 minutes, or until the squash can be easily pierced with a fork.
3. Allow the squash to cool slightly, then transfer it to a blender. Add the water and butter and blend until smooth, scraping down the sides as needed. Add water, if needed, until the desired consistency is reached.
4. Add the rosemary and blend until well incorporated.
5. Store leftovers in a sealed container in the refrigerator for up to 3 days or freeze for up to 3 months.

Tip: Fresh butternut squash can also be peeled, cubed, and steamed in a steamer basket or simmered in water for 15 minutes, or until tender. You can also roast a 1-pound butternut squash (which will make about 3 cups of puree): Simply slice the squash in half, scoop out the seeds, brush the flesh with melted butter, and roast cut-side down for 20 to 25 minutes at 375°F. Then, pick up the recipe at step 3 and proceed as instructed.

Rich Broccoli Puree

**MAKES
1½ CUPS**

**Prep time:
5 minutes**

**Cook time:
10 minutes**

Freezer-Friendly

Gluten-Free

Healthy Fats

Nut-Free

Quick and Easy

Vegetarian

It can be hard to find vegetables like broccoli or kale in the baby food aisle without sweet fruits added to mask their flavor. We recommend offering bitter vegetables individually so that baby can learn to accept this complex flavor. Preparing vegetables with fat is a great way to help baby absorb nutrients. If your little one doesn't love it right away, don't sweat it. Keep vegetables like broccoli, cauliflower, and kale in the rotation as your child grows.

2 cups broccoli florets, roughly chopped (about 1 large head)

1 tablespoon unsalted butter or coconut oil
¼ to ½ cup water

1. Cover the bottom of a medium saucepan with 2 to 3 inches of water and bring it to a simmer over medium heat.
2. Put the broccoli into a steamer basket or stainless-steel colander and set it over the simmering water. Steam until bright and tender, 5 to 7 minutes. Keep a close eye on it so it doesn't overcook (when it is overcooked it will turn an olive green color).
3. Put the broccoli into a blender along with the butter. Pour in ¼ cup water and blend, adding more water, 1 tablespoon at a time, as needed to reach the desired consistency. Allow to cool before serving.
4. Store leftovers in a sealed container in the refrigerator for up to 3 days or freeze for up to 3 months.

Tip: This recipe works well with other cruciferous vegetables such as cauliflower or Brussels sprouts.

Creamy Prune Whip

MAKES 1 CUP

Prep time:
15 minutes

Early Introduction

Freezer-Friendly

Gluten-Free

Healthy Fats

No-Cook

Nut-Free

Quick and Easy

Vegetarian

Constipation is an unfortunate side effect for some babies as they transition to solid foods. A focus on variety might be your best bet at preventing it, but you can also try including prunes in baby's diet. These antioxidant-rich dried fruits contain sorbitol along with a special compound called dihydroxyphenyl isatin, both of which have natural laxative properties. Prunes are also a great natural sweetener for yogurt and oatmeal.

6 prunes, soaked in warm water for 10 to 15 minutes

1 cup plain whole milk yogurt (regular or Greek-style)

1 to 2 teaspoons ground flaxseed (optional)

1. Drain the prunes, reserving some of the soaking water. In a blender, combine the yogurt, prunes, and flaxseed (if using). If necessary, add a bit of water from soaking the prunes to get a smooth texture.
2. Blend until smooth and serve.
3. Store leftovers in a sealed container in the refrigerator for up to 3 days or freeze for up to 3 months.

Tip: Try freezing this mixture in an ice-pop mold for a sweet, soothing treat for a teething baby.

Spiced Pear Puree

MAKES 1½ TO 2 CUPS

**Prep time:
5 minutes**

Dairy-Free

Freezer-Friendly

Gluten-Free

No-Cook

Nut-Free

Quick and Easy

Vegan

Babies love and recognize sweet tastes like fruit thanks to breast milk or formula, but that doesn't mean they won't learn to love other flavors as well. We recommend offering a wide variety, including the sweet, warm flavor of this fruit puree, right from the start. Before using any produce in baby food, wash it thoroughly with water and apply some elbow grease.

5 small ripe pears, peeled   **Dash ground cloves**
Dash ground cinnamon

1. Slice the pears into quarters, removing and discarding the seeds and cores.
2. Transfer the pears to a blender and add the cinnamon and cloves. Blend until smooth, adding a splash of water, if needed.
3. Refrigerate leftovers in a sealed container for up to 3 days or freeze for up to 3 months.

Tip: Pears are ready to eat when the neck feels soft when gentle pressure is applied. For a super-simple chunky puree, peel, core, and de-seed soft ripe pears and mash them with a fork before serving.

Nutty Sweet Potato Puree

MAKES 1 CUP

Prep time:
5 minutes

Cook time:
20 minutes

Dairy-Free

Early Introduction

Freezer-Friendly

Gluten-Free

Healthy Fats

Quick and Easy

Vegan

This recipe provides a simple and tasty way to introduce peanuts or tree nuts. We created the recipe with peanut butter, an important allergen to introduce early, but you can easily swap in almond or cashew butter, or even tahini. Based on the latest research, current recommendations are to introduce peanuts early and often. Try putting them in baby's meal rotation a few times a week for the most effective allergy prevention.

1 medium to large sweet potato (about 1 pound), peeled and diced into 1-inch chunks

1 to 2 teaspoons creamy nut butter (peanut, almond, or cashew) or tahini

1. Cover the bottom of a medium saucepan with 2 to 3 inches of water and bring it to a simmer over medium heat.
2. Put the sweet potato chunks into a steamer basket or stainless-steel colander and set it over the simmering water. Steam for 15 to 20 minutes, or until soft. Allow to cool slightly.
3. Combine the sweet potato and peanut butter in a blender along with enough water to make a smooth mixture. Alternatively, mash the sweet potato and peanut butter with a fork until combined.
4. Store leftovers in a sealed container in the refrigerator for up to 3 days or freeze for up to 3 months.

Tip: To have sweet potatoes on hand in a snap, we like to stick a few in the oven whenever we are cooking something else (e.g., baking muffins, roasting a chicken). Whole sweet potatoes take 45 to 50 minutes to bake and 35 to 40 minutes to steam. Dicing, as we have done in this recipe, speeds up the steaming time.

Spiced Apple Overnight Oats Puree

**MAKES
1½ CUPS**

Prep time:
5 minutes,
plus overnight
to soak

Cook time:
5 minutes

Nut-Free

Vegetarian

Soaking whole grains like oats is an age-old custom that allows the nutrients in the grain to be more easily digested, something that may be especially important for babies who are new to digesting complex carbohydrates. The apple cider vinegar in this recipe activates an enzyme that works to break down phytic acid, making the oats easier to digest and allowing for more absorption of the minerals present in them.

3 tablespoons old-
    fashioned rolled or
    quick-cooking oats
1 medium apple,
    peeled, cored, and
    roughly chopped
3 dates, pitted and
    roughly chopped

¼ cup water
⅔ cup whole milk
1 teaspoon apple
    cider vinegar
½ teaspoon ground
    cinnamon

1. In a small bowl with a lid or in a mason jar, combine all of the ingredients. Shake and refrigerate overnight.
2. Put the soaked overnight oats into a small saucepan and cook over medium heat for about 5 minutes, or until the apples have softened and the oats have thickened.
3. Allow the oats to cool slightly, then put the mixture in a blender and blend until the desired consistency is reached.
4. Refrigerate leftovers in a sealed container for up to 3 days.

Tip: To make a chunky puree, skip the blender and mash the apple chunks with a fork. Stir in 1 to 2 teaspoons peanut butter for allergy protection.

Lentil Puree with Turmeric and Ginger

**MAKES
1¼ CUPS**

**Cook time:
35 minutes**

Dairy-Free

Freezer-Friendly

Gluten-Free

Iron-Rich

Vegan

Lentils are one of the richest plant-based sources of iron and have a naturally soft texture when cooked, making them a staple beginner food for baby. This quick-cook method gets a delicious dish ready to eat in under 40 minutes. Mild in flavor, lentils provide a perfect base for introducing aromatic spices like ginger and turmeric. Top this puree with a dollop of whole milk yogurt and serve alongside vitamin C–rich butternut squash puree (see page 25) for extra iron absorption.

½ cup lentils, rinsed
1 cup water
¼ teaspoon ground turmeric

¼ teaspoon ground ginger, or 1 tablespoon grated fresh ginger
1 tablespoon coconut oil

1. In a medium saucepan, combine the lentils and water and bring to a boil over medium heat.
2. Cover and reduce the heat to medium-low, add the turmeric and ginger, then simmer for 30 minutes, or until the lentils are tender.
3. Remove from the heat and stir in the coconut oil until melted. Put the lentil mixture into a blender and puree until the desired consistency is reached.
4. Refrigerate leftovers in a sealed container for up to 3 days or freeze for up to 3 months.

Tip: Cooked lentils are very tender, so pureeing this recipe is optional. If you prefer to soak the lentils before cooking, which makes them easier to digest and cuts the cooking time in half, cover 1 cup lentils with about 2 cups water and soak for 2 to 3 hours, then drain, rinse, and begin at step 1.

Savory Beef with Sweet Potato and Thyme

MAKES 2 CUPS

Prep time:
5 minutes

Cook time:
30 minutes

Dairy-Free

Freezer-Friendly

Gluten-Free

Healthy Fats

Iron-Rich

Nut-Free

Among the rows and rows of fruit and vegetable pouches in the baby food aisle, we noticed a lack of high-quality protein options—where's the beef? Iron is one of the most important nutrients for brain development during this crucial time, and one of the best sources of iron is beef. It also provides zinc, fat, and protein, which quickly growing baby requires. This poaching method is versatile and can be used for other beef cuts as well as for pork or chicken.

1 (8-ounce) beef sirloin, roughly cut into cubes
2 cups water

1 medium sweet potato, peeled and roughly chopped
2 thyme sprigs, or 1 teaspoon dried thyme

1. In a medium saucepan over medium heat, combine the beef, water, sweet potato, and thyme and bring to a simmer. Reduce the heat to medium-low and continue to simmer, covered, for 20 to 30 minutes, or until fork-tender.
2. Discard the thyme sprigs and allow the ingredients to cool slightly. Remove any extra fat, cartilage, or bones from the beef. With a slotted spoon, transfer the beef and sweet potato to a blender with about ½ cup of the cooking water. Blend until smooth, adding more cooking water as needed.
3. Store leftovers in a sealed container in the refrigerator for up to 3 days or freeze for up to 3 months.

Simple Salmon Puree

Prep time:
5 minutes

Cook time:
5 minutes

Dairy-Free

Early Introduction

Freezer-Friendly

Gluten-Free

Healthy Fats

Nut-Free

Quick and Easy

Fish is one of the most underrated first foods for baby. Its natural melt-in-the-mouth texture is perfect for gumming. Aside from being a great source of easily absorbed iron and protein, it is also a major dietary source of docosahexaenoic acid (DHA), an omega-3 fatty acid that has become famous over the past decade for its role in cognitive development during pregnancy and early childhood. Emerging research has even linked fish consumption in kids to better sleep quality. This method can be used with other fish, such as arctic cod, tilapia, or haddock.

½ pound boneless, skinless salmon

⅔ cup water

½ lemon, sliced into rings or wedges, seeds removed

1. In a medium saucepan, combine the salmon, water, and lemon. Over medium heat, bring the liquid to a boil, then cover and reduce the heat to medium-low.
2. Simmer for about 5 minutes, or until the fish flakes easily and is cooked through.
3. Pour ¼ cup of cooking water from the saucepan into a blender. Add the fish and pulse, adding more cooking water as needed, until the desired consistency is reached. Alternatively, flake and mash the fish with a fork and serve as is for babies 6 months and up.
4. Refrigerate leftovers in a sealed container for up to 2 days or freeze for up to 3 months.

Tip: Boil and puree some quick-cooking vegetables, like chopped spinach or broccoli, along with the fish.

Simple Liver Puree

MAKES 2 CUPS

Prep time:
5 minutes

Cook time:
8 minutes

Dairy-Free

Freezer-Friendly

Gluten-Free

Healthy Fats

Iron-Rich

Nut-Free

Quick and Easy

Although it may not be the most popular food, liver is one of the most nutrient-packed ones available. Very few foods come close to its vitamin and mineral profile, and it is high in nutrients that are especially important for babies and toddlers. Liver doesn't need to be eaten all that often to reap the benefits. Aim to serve this superfood on its own or stirred into other purees only a few times a month.

2 tablespoons olive
  oil, divided
1 pound beef liver, sliced

2 cloves garlic, minced
¼ to ½ cup water

1. In a large cast-iron skillet, heat 1 tablespoon of olive oil over medium heat. Add half the liver and cook for 3 to 4 minutes, or until browned. Flip the liver and cook for an additional 3 to 4 minutes, or until browned on all sides and cooked through. Remove to a plate. Repeat with the remaining oil and liver.
2. Transfer the liver to a blender and add the garlic.
3. Pour ¼ cup of water into the pan and deglaze it by scraping up any browned bits with a metal spatula. Add the liquid from the deglazed pan to the blender with the garlic and liver and pulse until smooth, adding more water as needed. Alternatively, mash the liver with a fork.
4. Store leftovers in a sealed container in the refrigerator for up to 2 days or freeze for up to 3 months.

Tip: For extra mineral content, add a cube of the frozen liver puree to the Baby Bolognese sauce (page 140), meatballs, meatloaf, or chili.

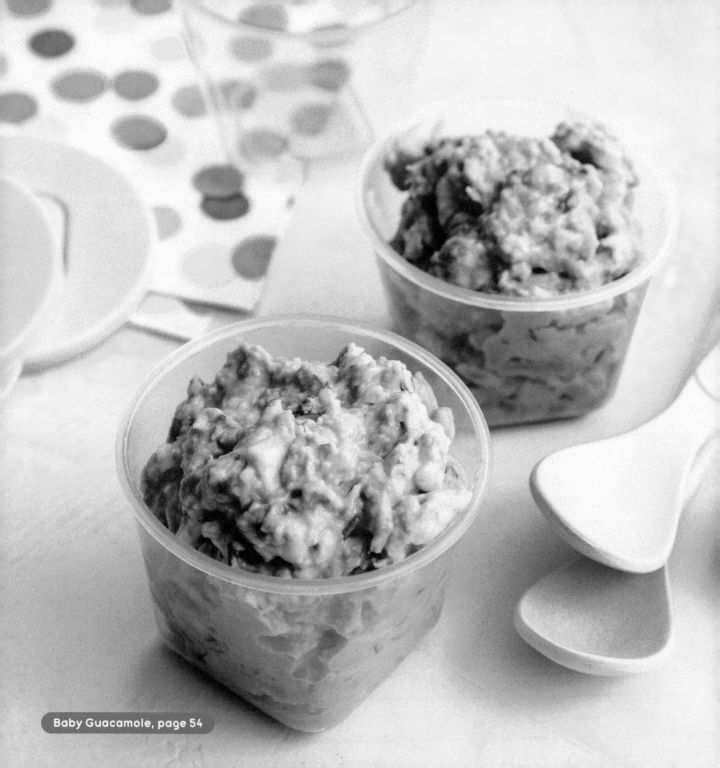

Baby Guacamole, page 54

CHAPTER 3

Chunky Purees
(6 to 12 Months)

In this chapter, we will continue to broaden the spectrum of flavors introduced to baby. We'll also showcase new textures and cooking methods to keep advancing their palates. Toasting, roasting, sautéing, and smashing each provide a unique mouthfeel for baby to master. Although some recipes still suggest blending, the majority have a naturally soft, chunky texture and can be eaten as is.

Along with introducing a wide variety of flavors and textures, remember to provide food in a responsive way by letting baby take the lead and following their cues for hunger and fullness, even if they aren't in control of the spoon quite yet.

Hearty Chicken Casserole

MAKES 1½ CUPS

Prep time:
10 minutes

Cook time:
25 minutes

Dairy-Free

Freezer-Friendly

Gluten-Free

Iron-Rich

Nut-Free

This nourishing chicken casserole recipe is the epitome of homemade comfort food. Rustic root vegetables like carrots and parsnips provide deep flavors alongside tender chicken breast and creamy potatoes. Though the leeks in this recipe are delicious, they can be easily replaced with an equal amount of chopped onion.

1 tablespoon olive oil
2 carrots, peeled and chopped
⅔ cup sliced leeks, white part only, washed
¼ pound boneless, skinless chicken breast, cut into 2-inch chunks

1 teaspoon chopped fresh herbs (such as rosemary, thyme, parsley, and/or sage)
2 potatoes, peeled and chopped
1 parsnip, peeled and chopped

1. In a medium saucepan, heat the olive oil over medium heat. Add the carrots and leeks. Sauté until the vegetables have softened, about 5 minutes. Add the chicken and herbs to the pan, sautéing for 5 to 7 minutes, or until the chicken is lightly browned and the internal temperature reaches 165°F.
2. Add the potatoes, parsnip, and enough water to just cover the contents of the pan. Cover and simmer for about 15 minutes, or until everything is fork-tender. Transfer all of the ingredients to a blender and puree until the desired consistency is reached, adding more water as necessary.
3. Store leftovers in a sealed container in the refrigerator for up to 3 days or freeze for up to 3 months.

Tip: If you stop just before blending in step 2, then others in the family can also enjoy this simple recipe. Or offer it lightly mashed for progressing older babies.

Caramelized Banana with Cinnamon

MAKES 1 CUP

Prep time:
2 minutes

Cook time:
6 minutes

Dairy-Free

Freezer-Friendly

Gluten-Free

Quick and Easy

Vegan

Bananas are one of the sweetest and most calorically dense fruits, making them an obvious kid favorite. Although ripe bananas can be simply mashed and served, this recipe offers a rich caramel flavor. Bananas are a versatile fruit for baby and can also be frozen and blended into a creamy treat with a texture similar to that of ice cream.

1 tablespoon coconut oil

2 bananas, sliced into rounds

½ teaspoon ground cinnamon

1. In a large cast-iron skillet, heat the coconut oil over medium heat until hot.
2. Add the banana slices in a single layer. Cook until golden brown, about 5 minutes. Flip the banana slices and cook for 2 to 3 minutes more. Remove from the heat.
3. Sprinkle the bananas with the cinnamon and mash with a fork until the desired consistency is reached. Allow to cool before serving.
4. Store leftovers in the refrigerator for up to 1 day or freeze for use in smoothies for up to 3 months (separation will occur after thawing).

Tip: For the rest of the family, this dish is delicious with whole milk yogurt and granola, or spread on top of almond butter toast. If you're in a time crunch, skip the caramelization (steps 1 and 2) and simply mash the uncooked banana with cinnamon for a similar flavor combination.

Dreamy Orange Chia Pudding

**Prep time:
10 minutes,
plus 2 to
3 hours to chill**

Dairy-Free

Gluten-Free

Healthy Fats

Iron-Rich

No-Cook

Vegan

Chia seeds are an amazing source of healthy fats, especially the omega-3 fatty acids that play such an important role in the brain development of little ones. They are also an excellent source of iron, which the vitamin C–rich orange juice helps little tummies absorb. Basically, chia seeds are an all-around powerhouse for babies (and grown-ups). The combo of coconut milk, orange juice, and chia makes this pudding creamy with a tapioca-like consistency that satisfies a sweet tooth. It's perfect for breakfast or a snack.

½ cup full-fat coconut milk
⅓ cup orange juice

1 teaspoon vanilla extract
3 tablespoons chia seeds

1. In a 12-ounce jar with a tight-fitting lid, combine the coconut milk, orange juice, and vanilla and shake until smooth.
2. Add the chia seeds, secure the lid, and shake to combine.
3. Refrigerate for at least 2 hours or up to overnight, until thickened.
4. Refrigerate leftovers in a sealed container for up to 2 days.

Tip: Mix and match other flavors with this pudding. As a general rule, 2 tablespoons of chia seeds require roughly ½ cup liquid to make a thick pudding. Try different add-ins, such as finely ground toasted nuts, pureed berries, or The Best Chunky Applesauce (page 56). Feel free to substitute whatever milk you have on hand for the coconut milk.

Tomato and Cauliflower Gratin

MAKES 1 CUP

Prep time:
5 minutes

Cook time:
15 minutes

Early Introduction

Gluten-Free

Healthy Fats

Nut-Free

Vegetarian

Although cauliflower was never invited to sit at the cool-kids' lunch table, it is one of our most favorite vegetables. A definite dinnertime underdog, cauliflower has an almost nutty flavor profile that transforms depending on the cooking method you use. We encourage caregivers to focus on flavor and nutrient profile over progression of textures. Bitter, sweet, sour, and umami—regularly include them all.

2 tablespoons unsalted butter
1 cup roughly
    chopped cauliflower

1 large tomato,
    roughly chopped
¼ cup shredded
    cheddar cheese

1. In a medium skillet, melt the butter over medium heat. Add the chopped cauliflower and sauté until tender, about 10 minutes.
2. Add the tomato and cook until soft, 2 to 3 minutes. Remove from the heat and stir in the grated cheese until melted.
3. Mash with a fork and serve.
4. Refrigerate leftovers in a sealed container for up to 3 days.

Tip: Other cruciferous vegetables like chopped broccoli or Brussels sprouts are delicious in this recipe as well.

Smashed Chickpea, Avocado, and Egg Salad

MAKES 2 CUPS

Prep time: 15 minutes, plus 1 hour to chill

Early Introduction

Gluten-Free

Healthy Fats

No-Cook

Nut-Free

Vegetarian

We realize we're technically in baby food territory here, but this recipe can very easily be served to the whole family. It is a twist on classic egg salad, featuring healthy fats, protein, and choline. Cilantro adds fresh flavor but can be omitted if you don't happen to have it on hand. Serve this salad on its own or spread on toasted bread.

1 ripe avocado, halved and pitted

1 teaspoon fresh lemon juice

4 tablespoons plain whole milk Greek yogurt

2 tablespoons chopped fresh cilantro (optional)

3 hard-boiled eggs, peeled and finely chopped

½ cup cooked or canned low-sodium chickpeas, drained and mashed with a fork

Freshly ground black pepper (optional)

1. Scoop the flesh of the avocado into a small bowl. Add the lemon juice and, using a fork, mash the avocado until it is fairly smooth and well combined with the lemon juice.
2. Add the yogurt and cilantro (if using) and mix well. Stir in the chopped hard-boiled eggs and mashed chickpeas and mix until combined.
3. Season with pepper (if using) and chill for at least 1 hour before serving.
4. Store leftovers in a sealed container in the refrigerator for up to 2 days.

Tip: Use the rest of the chickpeas in the can by adding them to a recipe in chapter 2 for a thicker, creamier puree that is easy for baby to self-feed.

Flaked Salmon with Mashed Potatoes

MAKES 1 CUP

Prep time:
10 minutes

Cook time:
15 minutes

Early Introduction

Freezer-Friendly

Gluten-Free

Healthy Fats

Iron-Rich

Nut-Free

Quick and Easy

A meal so tasty it invites the rest of the fam to join in! For this recipe, you can use fresh or canned salmon (bones removed). Some parents are surprised to hear that canned salmon is one of our whole food staples. Many of the options on the shelf are wild-caught and rich in omega-3 fatty acids (especially DHA) while being incredibly convenient and economical. Our kiddos have been known to eat it straight from the can!

2 medium yellow potatoes, peeled

3 tablespoons unsalted butter

2 tablespoons whole milk Greek yogurt

Freshly ground black pepper (optional)

½ cup flaked canned salmon, bones removed

1. Roughly cube the potatoes and put them into a small saucepan. Cover with water and bring to a boil over high heat. Cook until fork-tender, about 15 minutes. Remove from the heat.
2. Mash the hot potatoes with the butter and Greek yogurt until the desired consistency is reached. Season with pepper (if using).
3. Top the warm potatoes with the flaked salmon and serve.
4. Store leftovers in a sealed container in the refrigerator for up to 3 days or freeze for up to 3 months.

Tip: For a quick poached salmon recipe, see Simple Salmon Puree on page 33.

Roasted Apple and Acorn Squash Puree

MAKES 2 CUPS

Prep time:
5 minutes

Cook time:
50 minutes

Freezer-Friendly

Gluten-Free

Healthy Fats

Nut-Free

Vegetarian

We love a roast-and-go recipe. Rich in vitamin C, the acorn squash and apples offer impressive support for immune function. This dish pairs great with recipes that require a little more hands-on work like Aunt Marge's Classic Italian Meatballs (page 132).

1 acorn squash
2 apples, peeled, cored, and chopped
2 tablespoons unsalted butter, cut into small pieces

½ teaspoon ground cinnamon
½ teaspoon fresh or dried rosemary (optional)

1. Preheat the oven to 375°F.
2. Split the acorn squash in half and scoop out the seeds. Put the squash halves cut-side up on a rimmed baking sheet. Fill each half with the chopped apples and butter, then sprinkle with the cinnamon and rosemary (if using).
3. Roast for 45 to 50 minutes, or until the squash and apples are soft.
4. Allow to cool slightly, then scoop the squash and apples from the skin and transfer them to a blender. Discard the skin. Blend until the desired consistency is reached or, alternatively, mash the squash and apples with a fork.
5. Store leftovers in a sealed container in the refrigerator for up to 3 days or freeze for up to 3 months.

Tip: If you're short on time, you can cook the squash, apples, butter, and spices in a microwave-safe dish for 10 to 15 minutes, or until the flesh is tender. A butternut squash would be an excellent substitute when acorn squash is out of season.

Creamy Tomato and Chickpea Puree

MAKES 2 CUPS

Prep time:
5 minutes

Cook time:
20 minutes

Dairy-Free

Gluten-Free

Nut-Free

Quick and Easy

Vegan

Chickpeas give this classic tomato soup a thick and creamy texture that is easy for baby to scoop up themselves using a spoon or even their hands. Sounds messy, right? Letting little ones get their hands into their food helps them learn about it and become more comfortable with this whole eating-real-food thing. Drizzle a little cream or olive oil over the top before sprinkling with pepper, if desired, to add some extra healthy fats.

1 tablespoon olive oil
½ small onion, diced
2 garlic cloves, minced
1 (15-ounce) can diced
    or crushed tomatoes,
    no salt added
¼ cup water
1 cup cooked or canned
    low-sodium chickpeas,
    drained and rinsed

½ teaspoon dried oregano,
    or 1½ teaspoons chopped
    fresh oregano
½ teaspoon dried basil,
    or 1½ tablespoons
    chopped fresh basil
Freshly ground black
    pepper (optional)

1. Heat the oil in a medium Dutch oven or stockpot over medium heat. Add the onion and garlic and cook, stirring occasionally, for about 5 minutes, or until the onion has softened and the garlic is fragrant.
2. Pour in the tomatoes, water, chickpeas, oregano, and basil. Stir, then cover and simmer for about 15 minutes, or until heated through.

3. Using an immersion blender, blend until smooth. You can also blend the soup in batches in the blender or food processor.
4. Allow to cool slightly before serving. Lightly season with pepper (if using).
5. Store leftovers in a sealed container in the refrigerator for up to 3 days.

Tip: Make this a family meal by doubling the recipe. Older babies and other family members can also enjoy it with Creamy Avocado Grilled Cheese (page 70).

Pecan Coconut Skillet Oatmeal

**MAKES
2½ CUPS**

**Prep time:
5 minutes**

**Cook time:
10 minutes**

Early Introduction

Quick and Easy

Vegetarian

Nothing brings out the rich flavor of nuts like a good toasting. The warm aroma of toasting pecans and coconut will make the house smell like it's Christmas morning. Even better, the whole recipe can be cooked in the same cast-iron skillet, adding an extra punch of iron to the nutrient profile.

1 cup old-fashioned
   rolled oats
¼ cup chopped pecans
¼ cup unsweetened
   shredded coconut

1¼ cups whole milk, plus
   more as needed
1 teaspoon ground cinnamon

1. In a dry cast-iron skillet, spread out the oats, pecans, and shredded coconut evenly and toast over medium heat for 4 to 5 minutes, or until lightly browned and fragrant.
2. Put the toasted ingredients into a blender and pulse three or four times, or until the mixture has the texture of coarse sand.
3. Put the oat mixture back into the skillet, along with the milk and cinnamon. Stir and bring to a boil over medium-high heat, then reduce the heat to low, cover the skillet, and simmer, stirring occasionally, for 3 to 5 minutes, or until the mixture thickens. If the consistency is too thick, more milk can be added.
4. Remove from the heat and let cool before serving.

Tip: In a pinch for time? The toasting step can be skipped entirely, and the recipe can be prepared as traditional oatmeal by putting the untoasted oats, pecans, and coconut in the blender in step 2, then proceeding with the recipe as directed.

Black Bean Puree

MAKES 1½ CUPS

**Prep time:
5 minutes**

Dairy-Free

Freezer-Friendly

Gluten-Free

Iron-Rich

No-Cook

Quick and Easy

Nut-Free

Vegan

Black beans are one of our very favorite foods. We have even been known to make brownies with them. Packed with protein and iron, they are nutrient dense, filling, and hugely economical. We often prepare dried beans by soaking them overnight and cooking them on the stovetop, but we also love the convenience of canned beans. Look for "low sodium" or "no added sodium" on the label, or simply drain and rinse the canned beans before serving.

1 (15-ounce) can low-
    sodium black beans,
    drained and rinsed
2 tablespoons olive oil

2 tablespoons
    tahini (optional)
½ teaspoon ground cumin
Freshly ground black pepper

1. Combine the beans, olive oil, tahini (if using), cumin, and pepper in a blender and pulse a few times until well combined but still chunky. Alternately, mash the mixture with a fork until combined but still chunky.
2. Store leftovers in a sealed container in the refrigerator for up to 3 days or freeze for up to 3 months.

Tip: This chunky puree makes a great dip for the whole family. Spread it on strips of pita for older babies, or offer a bowl of it with crackers for an easy appetizer.

Garlicky Shrimp and Grits

SERVES 4

Prep:
5 minutes

Cook time:
15 minutes

Early Introduction

Iron-Rich

Nut-Free

Quick and Easy

Grits are a Southern mealtime staple that have a subtle corn flavor, making a hearty foundation for many meals. Whether served swimming in butter for breakfast or with a dash of Cajun spices at dinnertime, creamy grits have a great texture for young eaters and can be enjoyed by the whole family. The addition of shrimp in this recipe intentionally adds the shellfish allergen for introductory purposes, plus the naturally tender shrimp is perfect for first-time feeding.

2 cups water, plus
   more as needed
2 cups whole milk
4 tablespoons (½ stick)
   unsalted butter
½ teaspoon minced garlic
1 cup quick-cooking grits

1 cup shredded sharp
   cheddar cheese
1 tablespoon olive oil
1 pound raw shrimp,
   peeled and deveined
Freshly ground black
   pepper (optional)

1. In a large saucepan, bring the water, milk, butter, and garlic to a boil over medium-high heat. Slowly stir in the grits. Reduce the heat to medium, then cover and cook for 7 to 10 minutes, or until thickened.
2. When the consistency is smooth and most of the liquid is absorbed, stir in the cheese until melted. Add up to ½ cup more water, if necessary, to thin the consistency. Remove from the heat, set aside, and keep warm. (Grits will thicken upon cooling.)

3. In a medium skillet, heat the olive oil on medium-high and lay the shrimp flat in a single layer. Cook for 1 to 2 minutes, flip, and cook for another 1 to 2 minutes, or until they're pink and tender.

4. Transfer the shrimp to a cutting board and remove the tails (if still attached), then roughly chop to the desired size. Stir the shrimp pieces into the cheddar grits, add pepper if desired, and serve.

Tip: For self-feeding practice, the shrimp tails make a perfect little handle for holding, so just butterfly the meat for baby to enjoy! This recipe is one the whole family will love. For a quick flavor upgrade, add a dash of Cajun seasoning to the raw shrimp and sauté them with a few diced bell peppers and onions.

Chunky Split Pea Soup

**SERVES
4 TO 6**

**Prep time:
10 minutes**

**Cook time:
1 hour
10 minutes**

Dairy-Free

Freezer-Friendly

Gluten-Free

Nut-Free

Here's a fiber-filled, hearty soup that everyone in the family will enjoy! Slow cooking these rustic vegetables adds a delicious depth of flavor and makes them almost disappear within the soup, removing the need for additional pureeing for most eaters. Split peas are often overlooked in the grocery store, but their affordability and versatility make them a staple ingredient in a whole food kitchen.

2 quarts water
1 (16-ounce) bag dried split peas, rinsed (2¼ cups)
1 (1- to 2-pound) ham bone with some meat
2 onions, diced

½ teaspoon freshly ground black pepper
1 teaspoon dried marjoram
6 celery stalks, chopped
5 carrots, chopped
3 russet or golden potatoes, peeled and diced

1. In a large stockpot, combine the water and split peas over medium-high heat. When it comes to a boil, lower the heat to medium and simmer gently for 10 minutes, then turn off the heat, cover, and let the peas soak for about 10 minutes while you prep the other ingredients.
2. Uncover the pot and add the ham bone, onions, black pepper, marjoram, celery, carrots, and potatoes. Stir, then cover and bring to a boil over high heat. Reduce the heat to medium, then allow the soup to simmer for 45 to 60 minutes, stirring occasionally. All vegetables should be fork-tender and cooked down until most of the moisture is absorbed and the soup resembles a very thick and chunky puree.

3. Carefully transfer the bone from the pot to a cutting board, cut off any good meat, and discard the bone. Dice up the meat, then stir it back into the soup. If necessary, simmer uncovered until the desired thickness is reached.

4. Store leftovers in a sealed container in the refrigerator for up to 3 days or freeze for up to 3 months.

Tip: This recipe is the perfect solution for using up leftover bone-in ham, but you can easily swap in 1 to 2 cups diced ham if you have it on hand.

Baby Guacamole

MAKES ½ CUP

**Prep time:
5 minutes**

Gluten-Free

Healthy Fats

No-Cook

Nut-Free

Quick and Easy

Vegetarian

Squishy green avocado cheeks and fingers are definitely in our top-five favorite things. With heart-healthy fats, brain-building omega-3s, and a naturally soft texture, avocado is a baby food trifecta. The secret to good guac is a perfectly ripe avocado. Gently press on the neck (the skin close to the top stem), and if it gives slightly, then the avocado is ready to go. If not, set it in a window to ripen for another day.

1 small ripe avocado,
   halved and pitted
1 teaspoon minced fresh
   cilantro (optional)

1 tablespoon plain
   whole milk yogurt
1 lime

1. Scoop out the avocado flesh and put it into a small bowl. Discard the avocado skins. Add the cilantro (if using) and yogurt to the avocado.
2. Using a fork or potato masher, smash and mix until a chunky puree texture is achieved.
3. Give the lime a quick roll on the countertop, then halve it and squeeze the juice of one half over the mixture (reserve the remaining half for another use). Stir, then serve with a spoon as a dip for veggies, spread onto toast, or add a dollop to scrambled eggs.

Tip: Avocado does not freeze well, so you can always halve the recipe and save the remaining avocado for another day. Or if you want to refrigerate leftovers, you can prevent some discoloration by squeezing the lime juice over the top of the avocado without stirring it in and store in a tightly covered container. Who are we kidding—leftovers? Just stir in some diced onion, tomato, cumin, and cayenne and guac on!

Peach Sauce with Greek Yogurt

MAKES 1 CUP PEACH SAUCE

Prep time:
5 minutes

Cook time:
5 minutes

Early Introduction

Freezer-Friendly

Gluten-Free

Nut-Free

Quick and Easy

Vegetarian

Every morning in the late spring, Laura's toddlers race outside to check the progress of the peach trees growing in the yard. They occasionally even pull a tiny green peach off of a branch to sample. Fresh peaches are a signifier that summer has truly arrived, and this recipe is a great way to celebrate seasonal produce with little ones.

1 tablespoon unsalted butter
4 peaches, peeled, pitted, and diced (about 2½ cups)

½ teaspoon ground cinnamon
1 cup whole milk Greek yogurt, plain or vanilla

1. In a medium skillet or saucepan, melt the butter over medium heat. Add the peaches, sprinkle with the cinnamon, and sauté for about 5 minutes, or until soft, smashing the peaches with a wooden spatula while cooking. Remove from the heat.
2. Allow the peaches to cool until just warm and spoon them over the Greek yogurt.
3. Store leftovers in a sealed container in the refrigerator for up to 2 days or freeze the sauce (not the yogurt) for up to 3 months.

Tip: Toss leftover peach sauce into a smoothie or stir it into oatmeal.

The Best Chunky Applesauce

**MAKES
1½ CUPS**

Prep time:
10 minutes

Cook time:
25 minutes

Freezer-Friendly

Gluten-Free

Healthy Fats

Nut-Free

Vegetarian

What makes this applesauce different is its rich, caramel flavor. In most of our recipes for baby, you might notice we incorporate some fat. That's intentional because babies need about 50 percent of their daily calories from fat to support rapid body and brain development. Not to mention fat makes fruits and veggies taste even more delicious!

2 tablespoons unsalted butter
4 apples, peeled, cored,
  and chopped

½ teaspoon ground cinnamon
½ teaspoon vanilla extract

1. In a large cast-iron skillet over medium heat, melt the butter and swirl to coat the pan. Add the apples and cinnamon and cook, covered, for 10 minutes. Remove the cover and cook, stirring and flipping the apples every few minutes, for an additional 10 to 15 minutes, or until lightly browned.
2. Allow the apples to cool slightly, then either combine the apples and vanilla in the blender, pulsing a few times, or mash the apples and vanilla together with a fork until the desired consistency is reached.
3. Refrigerate leftovers in a sealed container for up to 3 days or freeze for up to 3 months.

Tip: Serve applesauce over plain whole milk yogurt or as a topping for Apple Sweet Potato Pancakes (page 62).

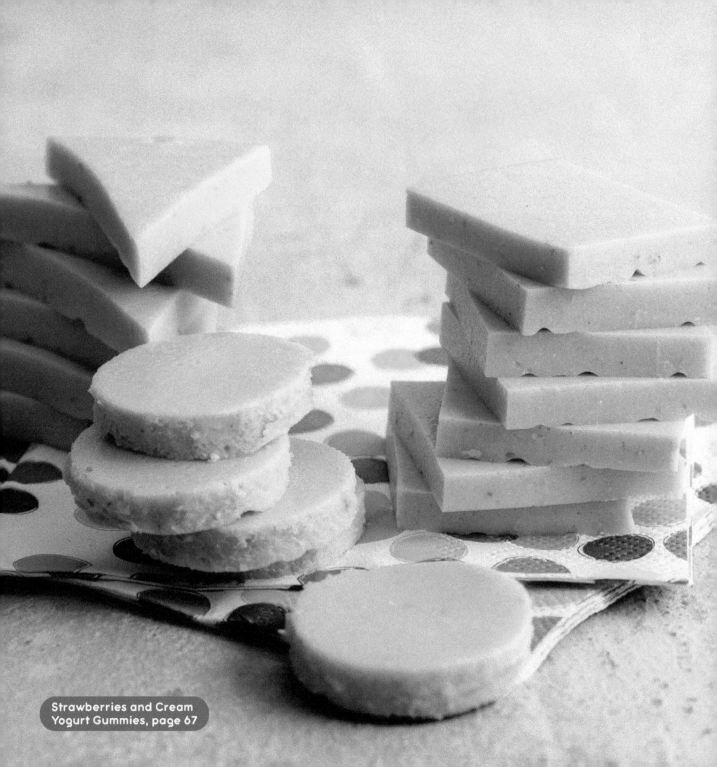

Strawberries and Cream
Yogurt Gummies, page 67

CHAPTER 4
Finger Food Firsts
(8 to 10 Months and Up)

It's time to dig in—hands first! Babies are such curious little creatures and are eager to get their hands into anything they can. So let's let them! The recipes in this section are simple to prepare and designed for easy pickup to encourage self-feeding. The bonus is these recipes taste great for the rest of the family, too!

We have chosen these recipes to focus on key nutrients needed for brain and body development during this time, like choline, DHA, vitamin A, B_{12}, and iron; baby will eat up this learning opportunity.

During this stage, do your best to sit back and let baby lead. Give them the opportunity to practice their new skills and watch in awe just how quickly they progress from clumsy little eaters to confident self-feeders. You'll see progression from a palmar to pincer grasp, and perhaps to dipping or scooping with utensils. Appetites can vary from day to day, so watch closely during mealtime to stay in tune with their cues of hunger and fullness. Becoming familiar with this appetite ebb and flow can help avoid mealtime frustrations.

Rainbow Fruit Salad

**Prep time:
10 to
15 minutes,
plus 1 hour
to chill**

Dairy-Free

Gluten-Free

No-Cook

Nut-Free

Vegan

Think of this recipe as a guide rather than a set of instructions to follow. For produce, we try to shop local and in-season as much as possible, so absolutely swap out any of these fruits for whatever your community has to offer. For a beautiful presentation and conversation stimulator at mealtimes, aim for at least one fruit from each color group.

1 pint strawberries (about 2 cups), sliced

1 (15-ounce) can mandarin oranges in light syrup, drained and rinsed

½ cup cubed pineapple

1 kiwi, peeled and sliced

½ pint blueberries (about 1 cup)

½ cup seedless grapes, quartered

1 cup cubed seedless watermelon

1 lemon or lime

1 banana

1. In a large bowl, combine all the fruits except the lemon and banana.
2. Roll the lemon on the countertop to tenderize the flesh and juice, then cut it in half and squeeze the juice over the fruit. Chill in the refrigerator for about 1 hour.
3. Just before serving, cut the banana into small chunks and gently stir it in.
4. Refrigerate leftovers in a sealed container for up to 3 days.

Tip: Kids in the kitchen is such an important concept. With simple template recipes like this, let them help; older children can choose a fruit from each color of the rainbow. Younger ones can roll the lemons and then, after removing the seeds, squeeze the juice over the top!

Apple Sweet Potato Pancakes

Prep time:
5 minutes

Cook time:
20 minutes

Early Introduction

Freezer-Friendly

Gluten-Free

On the Go

Quick and Easy

Vegetarian

These are a fresh, veggie-packed alternative to traditional breakfast pancakes, but we love them for any meal of the day. At home, spread butter over them or take them on the go with yogurt for dipping. The grated apple and sweet potato hold a lot of moisture, so laying them out on paper towels before mixing up the batter is a crucial step to ensure the pancakes hold together in the skillet.

1 medium apple, peeled and cored

1 large sweet potato, peeled

2 tablespoons unsalted butter, divided

2 eggs

½ teaspoon ground cinnamon

1. Using a box grater or food processor, grate the apple and sweet potato. Spread the shredded potato and apple onto paper towels or a clean dish towel and squeeze to remove excess moisture.
2. Melt 1 tablespoon of butter in a large cast-iron skillet over medium heat.
3. Meanwhile, in a medium bowl, combine the sweet potato, apple, eggs, and cinnamon. Stir well, making sure the egg evenly coats the potato mixture.
4. Pour in about ½ cup of the mixture into the hot skillet. Spread it out to flatten it, keeping the mixture as densely packed as possible so the pancake isn't too thin to hold together. Cook for 3 to 4 minutes, or until browned and crispy. Flip and cook on the other side for 3 to 4 minutes more. Repeat with the remaining batter, using the remaining 1 tablespoon of butter as necessary.
5. Refrigerate leftovers in a sealed container for up to 2 days or freeze for up to 3 months.

Two-Ingredient Pancakes

MAKES 6 TO 8 SMALL (2-INCH) PANCAKES

Prep time:
5 minutes

Cook time:
5 minutes

Early Introduction

Freezer-Friendly

Gluten-Free

Healthy Fats

Nut-Free

On the Go

Quick and Easy

Vegetarian

With just two ingredients, pancakes don't get any easier. This recipe can be doubled to make extra pancakes for the freezer, and as baby grows and their tastes develop, feel free to stir in any of the following to vary the flavors and texture: cinnamon, vanilla, fresh berries, granola, or cocoa.

1 ripe banana
2 large eggs, lightly beaten

1 tablespoon unsalted butter, for greasing the pan

1. In a medium bowl, mash the banana until it has a pudding-like consistency.
2. Stir in the eggs until completely incorporated.
3. Heat a medium skillet over medium heat. Put the butter into the pan, and when it begins to sizzle, drop about 2 tablespoons of batter on the hot skillet for each pancake. (The batter should begin to sizzle immediately.) Repeat until the pan is filled, leaving 1 to 2 inches between each pancake.
4. Cook for about 1 minute. The corners should be set, and when you peek at the underside, it should be golden brown. Carefully flip the pancakes and cook for about 1 minute more, or until browned.
5. Serve warm with the topping of your choice, like butter, peanut butter, or maple syrup.
6. Store leftovers in a sealed container in the refrigerator for up to 3 days or in the freezer for up to 3 months.

Skillet-Fried Green Peas

MAKES 1 CUP

Prep time:
5 minutes

Cook time:
10 minutes

Gluten-Free

Healthy Fats

Nut-Free

On the Go

Quick and Easy

Vegetarian

These crunchy peas are perfect for little learning fingers. In our families, the kitchen is our classroom, and simple recipes like this make a delicious tool for practicing baby's pincer grasp. Pinching and moving food from plate to mouth is a skill babies will literally use the rest of their lives.

1 tablespoon unsalted butter   **1 cup frozen green peas**
1 teaspoon minced garlic

1. In a large cast-iron skillet, melt the butter over medium heat. Add the garlic and green peas.
2. Cook for 5 to 7 minutes, or until the peas are browned and a little crispy.
3. Remove from the heat and enjoy.
4. Store leftovers in a sealed container in the refrigerator for up to 3 days.

Tip: This cooking method can be used as a tasty alternative to steaming or boiling any frozen vegetable, including broccoli florets, green beans, mixed vegetables, lima beans, corn, and spinach.

Black Bean–Sweet Potato Burgers

MAKES 12 TO 14 (2-INCH) MINI PATTIES

Prep time:
15 minutes

Cook time:
25 minutes

Dairy-Free

Freezer-Friendly

Iron-Rich

Nut-Free

On the Go

Vegetarian

These flavor-packed burgers can be served whole or sliced into strips as soon as your little one is showing interest in self-feeding. Pair iron-rich foods like beans with those high in vitamin C to increase iron absorption. This is especially important when it comes to plant-based iron.

1 medium sweet potato, cooked and flesh scooped from skin

1 cup cooked or canned low-sodium black beans, drained and rinsed

1 egg, lightly beaten

⅓ cup panko bread crumbs

⅓ cup old-fashioned rolled oats

½ teaspoon ground cumin

Freshly ground black pepper

2 to 3 tablespoons olive oil

1. Line a large plate with parchment paper.
2. In a large bowl, mash the sweet potato and black beans with a fork until combined. Add the egg, then add the bread crumbs, oats, cumin, and black pepper to taste and stir until well combined.
3. Using about ¼ cup of the mixture for each, form small patties using your clean hands (this part can be a little messy). Place the patties on the prepared plate.
4. In a large cast-iron skillet, heat 2 tablespoons of olive oil over medium heat. When it is hot, place half of the patties in the pan and cook until golden brown, about 5 to 6 minutes. Flip and cook for 5 to 6 minutes more. Repeat with the remaining patties, adding more oil if needed.
5. Store leftovers in a sealed container in the refrigerator for up to 2 days or freeze for up to 3 months.

Mini Oyster Fritters

MAKES 5 OR 6 (2-INCH) MINI FRITTERS

Prep time:
10 minutes

Cook time:
10 minutes

Dairy-Free

Early Introduction

Freezer-Friendly

Iron-Rich

Nut-Free

On the Go

Quick and Easy

Cooked oysters are another one of the most nutrient-dense foods on the planet. Like liver, they are a great source of nutrients that are of particular importance to babies and toddlers: iron, zinc, vitamin B_{12}, and vitamin D in addition to omega-3 fatty acids. They are found canned most often and are very tender, making chopped oysters a great snack for little ones. Look for "non-BPA liner" printed on the can before buying, if possible.

2 (3-ounce) cans oysters, drained, rinsed, and finely chopped

½ cup panko bread crumbs

1 egg

1 tablespoon fresh lemon juice

¼ cup chopped fresh parsley, or 1 teaspoon dried parsley

½ teaspoon garlic powder

2 to 3 tablespoons olive oil

1. In a medium mixing bowl, combine the oysters, bread crumbs, egg, lemon juice, parsley, and garlic powder and mix well. Then, with clean hands, form the mixture into small 2-inch patties.
2. In a large cast-iron skillet, heat the oil over medium heat. Swirl the pan to cover the bottom and sides of the pan with oil, then fry the patties for 3 to 5 minutes on each side. When the patties have cooked, transfer them to a plate and set aside to cool.
3. Serve the fritters whole, sliced into strips, or cut into bite-size pieces.
4. Store leftovers in the refrigerator for up to 2 days or freeze for up to 3 months.

Strawberries and Cream Yogurt Gummies

**Prep time:
15 minutes,
plus 2 hours
15 minutes to
cool and set**

**Cook time:
10 minutes**

Gluten-Free

Healthy Fats

Nut-Free

On the Go

Aside from being jiggly, pink, and all around kid-friendly, homemade gummies are surprisingly healthy. Gelatin is derived from majorly trendy collagen, which is rich in high-quality protein that may reverse tummy troubles such as diarrhea or constipation. Some studies even show an increase in quality of sleep thanks to the jiggly stuff! You can find unflavored gelatin packets in the baking aisle of the grocery store.

1 cup cold whole milk

4 (¼-ounce) packets (about 2¼ teaspoons each) gelatin

2 cups frozen strawberries, thawed

½ cup vanilla whole milk Greek yogurt

1 teaspoon vanilla extract

1. Line a 9-by-13-inch baking dish with parchment paper.
2. In a small bowl, combine the milk and gelatin. Whisk and allow it to sit for 5 minutes, until thickened.
3. Combine the berries, yogurt, and vanilla in a blender and blend until smooth.
4. Pour the pureed berry mixture into a medium saucepan and heat it over medium heat until hot but not boiling, about 7 minutes. Add the gelatin/milk mixture and whisk until well combined.
5. Remove the pan from the heat and let cool for 15 minutes. Pour it into the prepared baking dish, cover, and refrigerate until set, about 2 hours.
6. Cut into small squares or use a cookie cutter to create fun shapes.
7. Store leftovers in a sealed container in the refrigerator for up to 2 days.

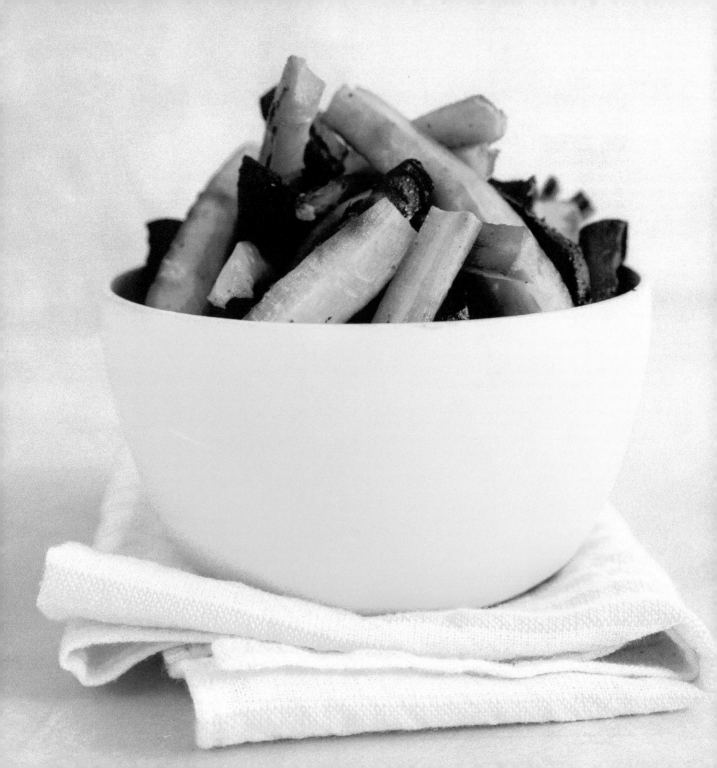

Maple Roasted Beet and Carrot Fries

SERVES 4

Prep time:
10 minutes

Cook time:
20 minutes

Dairy-Free

Gluten-Free

Healthy Fats

Nut-Free

Quick and Easy

Vegan

Every year in July, Laura's family runs into a familiar dilemma: what to do with way too many beets from the garden. Beets are great for adding color and variety, but they tend to taste a little, uhm, earthy. Roasting beets and carrots with a touch of maple syrup brings out the natural sweetness of both vegetables, making them a dinnertime fave (even for little ones claiming they don't like "beeps").

3 medium beets, scrubbed
   and greens removed
4 large carrots
2 tablespoons olive oil

2 tablespoons maple syrup
Freshly ground black
   pepper (optional)

1. Preheat the oven to 425°F. Line a rimmed baking sheet with parchment paper.
2. Slice the beets into rounds and then into ½-inch matchsticks. Slice the carrots in half lengthwise, then in half crosswise, then into ½-inch matchsticks. Spread the beets and carrots on the prepared baking sheet.
3. In a small bowl, whisk together the olive oil and maple syrup. Pour the mixture over the beet and carrot fries and toss to coat. Arrange in a single layer. Sprinkle with pepper, if using.
4. Roast the beet and carrot fries for 15 to 20 minutes, until fork-tender, flipping halfway through.
5. Refrigerate leftovers in a sealed container for up to 2 days.

Tip: Although many recipes advise peeling carrots and beets, you don't have to peel them to get great results. In addition, many fruits and veggies retain a lot of nutrients in the skins. Beets are especially hard to peel, and you can hardly tell the difference once they are roasted.

Creamy Avocado Grilled Cheese

**MAKES
1 SANDWICH**

**Prep time:
5 minutes**

**Cook time:
10 minutes**

Healthy Fats

Nut-Free

On the Go

Quick and Easy

Vegetarian

When choosing bread, the most important factor from a whole food perspective is a short ingredients list. Store-bought bread can be a hiding place for a lot of added sugar, salt, and synthetic additives. Although homemade bread is delicious, it isn't always practical (though we do attempt it every now and then). Choose a bread your family enjoys that is made with real, easy-to-identify ingredients like whole wheat, water, a leavening agent, and salt.

2 slices bread
1 tablespoon unsalted butter, at room temperature

½ ripe avocado, peeled and mashed
2 ounces shredded cheddar cheese (about ½ cup)

1. Heat a medium cast-iron skillet over medium heat.
2. Spread one side of each bread slice with butter. Place one slice of bread buttered-side down in the skillet.
3. Spread the avocado on the slice in the skillet and top it with the cheese and the remaining slice of bread, buttered-side up. Cook for about 5 minutes, or until the bottom side of the bread is golden brown, then flip and cook on the other side for 3 to 5 minutes, until the bread is golden brown and the cheese has melted.
4. Transfer the sandwich to a cutting board and allow it to cool before slicing it into strips or wedges for baby.

Tip: Pair this sandwich with Creamy Tomato and Chickpea Puree (page 46).

Whole Food Teething Biscuits

MAKES 24 BISCUITS

Prep time:
10 minutes

Cook time:
20 minutes

Early Introduction

Freezer-Friendly

Healthy Fats

On the Go

Quick and Easy

Vegetarian

Teething biscuits aren't a necessary part of baby's diet, as there are plenty of whole food options for teething babies to gum on, like sticks of celery, cucumber, cold watermelon, or homemade ice pops. However, a lot of busy families are looking for snacks that can be taken on the road, and they often opt for processed snacks marketed for babies. This nutrient-dense recipe fulfills the same role while being much cheaper *and* healthier.

3 cups old-fashioned
    rolled oats
1 cup pecan or walnut halves
1 teaspoon ground cinnamon
1 ripe banana

¼ cup peeled and mashed
    cooked sweet potato
    or butternut squash
5 tablespoons unsalted
    butter, melted

1. Preheat the oven to 350°F. Line a rimmed baking sheet with parchment paper.
2. In a food processor or blender, pulse the oats and pecans until fine crumbs form. Add the cinnamon and pulse once to combine.
3. In a medium mixing bowl, mash the banana and sweet potato together, stir in the butter, and mix until well combined. Add the oat mixture and stir just until incorporated.
4. Form about 2 tablespoons of oat mixture into a ball and place it on the prepared baking sheet. Press down on top gently to flatten it. Repeat with the remaining dough.
5. Bake for 20 minutes, or until golden brown and crispy.
6. Refrigerate leftovers in a sealed container for up to 2 days or freeze for up to 3 months.

Cheesy Zucchini Bites

MAKES 8 TO 10 SMALL (2-INCH) FRITTERS

Prep time:
10 minutes

Cook time:
25 minutes

Early Introduction

Freezer-Friendly

Healthy Fats

Nut-Free

Vegetarian

Crispy, cheesy bites of veggie-packed goodness are a great way to sum up this recipe. Little ones like them dipped in ketchup, whereas the grown-ups in the house can use them as a salad topper or delicious side for any meal. They are even "snacky" enough to be eaten as an appetizer or during the big game. The mixture may feel a little wet when forming the bites, but they will bake up crispy as long as any excess moisture has been removed from the zucchini.

1½ cups shredded zucchini (about 1 medium zucchini)
2 eggs
½ cup shredded cheddar cheese (about 2 ounces)
¼ cup panko bread crumbs
½ teaspoon garlic powder
1 tablespoon chopped fresh basil, or 1 teaspoon dried basil
2 tablespoons olive oil

1. Preheat the oven to 350°F. Line a rimmed baking sheet with parchment paper.
2. Spread the shredded zucchini on a clean dish towel or paper towels and squeeze to remove any excess moisture.
3. In a medium mixing bowl, combine the zucchini, eggs, cheese, bread crumbs, garlic powder, and basil and mix well.
4. Scooping up 2 to 3 tablespoons at a time, form the batter into patties with your clean hands.
5. Place each patty on the prepared baking sheet and drizzle with the olive oil. Bake for 25 minutes, or until golden brown on the bottom.
6. Refrigerate leftovers in a sealed container for up to 2 days or freeze for up to 3 months.

Veggie-Packed Beef and Quinoa Meatloaf

**SERVES
4 TO 6**

**Prep time:
15 minutes**

**Cook time:
1 hour**

Dairy-Free

Freezer-Friendly

Iron-Rich

Nut-Free

We love to add whole grains to recipes with ground meat whenever possible. It not only helps with the family food budget but also adds nutrients such as fiber and B vitamins. The result is a budget-friendly, flavorful meatloaf that also sneaks in an extra serving of vegetables.

1 tablespoon olive oil
1 onion, finely chopped
2 garlic cloves, minced
2 carrots, grated
2½ cups chopped
   fresh spinach
1 pound ground beef

1 cup cooked quinoa
1 egg, lightly beaten
2 tablespoons low-
   sodium soy sauce
¼ cup ketchup or
   barbecue sauce

1. Preheat the oven to 425°F. Line a rimmed baking sheet with parchment paper.
2. Heat the oil in a large cast-iron skillet over medium heat. Add the onion, garlic, and carrots and sauté for 5 to 7 minutes, or until softened. Add the spinach and sauté for 2 to 3 minutes more, or until just wilted. Set aside to cool slightly.
3. In a large mixing bowl, combine the sautéed vegetables, beef, quinoa, egg, and soy sauce and mix well (you might need to use your hands).
4. Transfer the mixture to the prepared baking sheet and form into a loaf using your clean hands. Top with the ketchup and bake for 45 minutes, or until browned and the internal temperature reaches 160°F. Allow to cool before serving.

Sweet Potato Cinnamon Muffins

MAKES 12 MUFFINS

Prep time:
15 minutes

Cook time:
25 minutes

Freezer-Friendly

On the Go

Vegetarian

Everybody needs a good muffin recipe in their back pocket for playdates, preschool snacks, or late Sunday morning breakfasts. Sweet Potato Cinnamon Muffins are just that!

Unsalted butter, for greasing

1 cup peeled and mashed cooked sweet potato

¼ cup packed dark brown sugar

¼ cup coconut oil, melted

½ cup whole milk

2 large eggs

1 teaspoon vanilla extract

1 cup old-fashioned rolled oats

1 cup unbleached all-purpose flour, or ½ cup whole wheat flour plus ½ cup unbleached all-purpose flour

1 teaspoon ground cinnamon, plus more (optional) for sprinkling

½ teaspoon pumpkin pie spice

2 teaspoons baking powder

1. Preheat the oven to 350°F.
2. Heat the muffin tin in the oven. When it's warm, remove it from the oven and carefully and thoroughly grease each muffin cup with butter.
3. In a large bowl, whisk together the mashed sweet potato, brown sugar, coconut oil, milk, eggs, and vanilla. Stir in the oats and flour. Mix until thoroughly incorporated.
4. Stir in the cinnamon, pumpkin pie spice, and baking powder. Fill each of the muffin cups two-third full with batter.

5. Sprinkle the tops of each muffin with additional cinnamon, if desired.
6. Bake for 22 to 25 minutes, or until the muffins begin to pull away from the sides and a toothpick inserted into the center of a muffin comes out clean.
7. Store leftovers in a sealed container in the refrigerator for up to 3 days or freeze for up to 3 months.
8. Store leftovers in a sealed container in the refrigerator for up to 3 days or freeze for up to 3 months.

Tip: Sweet potatoes are an incredibly versatile whole food that can be used in both sweet and savory recipes like pancakes, muffins, omelets—you name it!

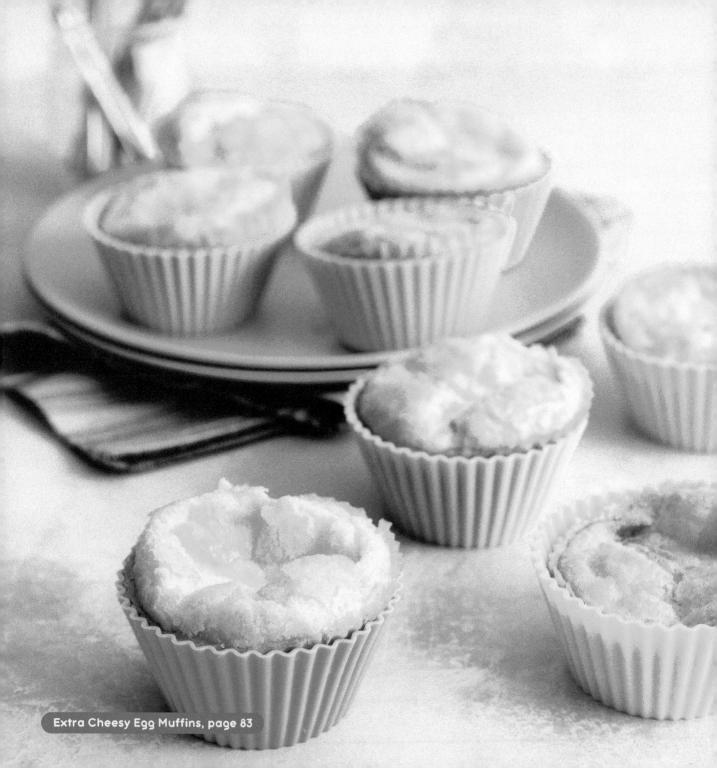

Extra Cheesy Egg Muffins, page 83

CHAPTER 5

Breakfast and Snacks
(12 Months and Up)

Big milestones are coming your way in this recipe section: the long awaited first birthday—don't worry, we've got the cake covered—big-kid breakfast ideas, and snack time solutions, along with simple family staples you'll wonder why you've never made before. Mealtimes and snacks should focus on variety. Your child's taste preferences may seem to be changing almost daily, so keep the kitchen fresh with new recipes to try. From now into toddlerhood, the foundation of an infant's diet will slowly be progressing away from breast milk or formula and transitioning into the majority of nutrients coming from table foods.

After one year, most foods are safe to offer baby, but use discretion with added sugars and salt from processed foods and cook with a scant amount of both. During this time, we want to focus on fostering independence at the table, self-feeding with hands or utensils, independently drinking from straws or sippy cups, practicing intuitive eating by stopping when full, and engaging with the rest of the family during mealtimes. Baby's all grown up!

Ricotta Cheese Breakfast Bowl

SERVES 2

**Prep time:
5 minutes**

Gluten-Free

Healthy Fats

No-Cook

Quick and Easy

Vegetarian

Let's be real. Some days you wake up more tired than when you went to bed and just don't feel like cooking. But the little ones are still hungry. For days like this, we like to keep a couple of no-cook meals in our back pocket. This breakfast bowl can be prepped and served before your brain knows it's awake.

½ cup whole milk
    ricotta cheese
2 tablespoons whole milk
2 tablespoons finely
    chopped almonds

2 tablespoons unsweetened
    flaked coconut
1 cup blueberries or fruit
    of your choice

In a small bowl, combine the ricotta and milk. Divide this mixture between 2 bowls. Sprinkle each with almonds and coconut. Top both with blueberries and serve.

Tip: If ricotta cheese is not a refrigerator staple in your home, classic cottage cheese makes a great substitution that also adds an extra blast of protein.

Yogurt Three Ways

MAKES ABOUT 1 CUP EACH

Prep time: 10 minutes each

Gluten-Free

Healthy Fats

Nut-Free

Quick and Easy

Vegetarian

Yogurt is one of those healthy whole foods that can easily be overprocessed. It is also one of the foods most likely to have a ton of health claims to cover up the multitude of added ingredients—this is especially true in yogurt products marketed to kids. To avoid the extras, your best bet is choosing plain whole milk yogurt and flavoring it yourself at home. We even include a savory option!

Date Caramel

1 (8-ounce) bag pitted dates
¼ cup hot water, plus
   more as needed

1 cup plain whole milk yogurt
   (Greek or regular)

1. Put the dates and ¼ cup hot water in the bowl of a food processor. Pulse until a smooth paste forms, adding more water as needed to achieve this texture.
2. Stir 1 to 2 teaspoons of the date caramel into the plain yogurt before serving.
3. Store the date caramel in a sealed container in the refrigerator for up to 2 weeks.

Chia Jam

4 cups fresh or frozen berries
1 tablespoon maple syrup
¼ cup chia seeds, plus
   more as needed

1 cup plain whole milk yogurt
   (Greek or regular)

1. In a large saucepan over medium heat, cook the berries for about 10 minutes (no need to thaw if frozen, but allow frozen berries to cook longer).

2. Remove from the heat and mash the berries with a fork or transfer them to a blender and blend until a sauce forms. Stir in the maple syrup and chia seeds.
3. Pour the berry sauce into a pint-size jar with a tight-fitting lid and allow it to cool and thicken (about 2 minutes). If you would like a thicker consistency, add an additional teaspoon of chia seeds.
4. Stir 1 to 2 tablespoons of the chia jam into plain yogurt before serving.
5. Store the chia jam in the refrigerator for up to 1 week (the mixture will continue to thicken in the refrigerator) or freeze for up to 3 months.

Tip: For a smoother texture, place the thickened jam in a blender and blend until smooth. It can also be spread on toast, stirred into oatmeal, or blended into smoothies.

Taco Dip

2 tablespoons salsa
2 tablespoons shredded cheddar cheese

1 cup plain whole milk yogurt (Greek or regular)

1. In a small mixing bowl, combine the salsa, shredded cheese, and yogurt. Mix well and serve immediately or chill before serving.
2. Store in a sealed container in the refrigerator for up to 3 days.

Happy Toddler Smoothie

When older babies and toddlers enter a picky phase (as they almost always do), we recommend continuing business as usual by offering a wide variety of foods until the phase passes. We also know that it can be stressful to see our little one refuse foods they used to eat happily, and many parents consider a toddler formula or nutrition shake. This smoothie packs in as many calories as store-bought toddler nutrition drinks (one 4-ounce serving has about 120 calories) without all of the additives and sugar.

1 cup whole milk or kefir
½ cup whole milk yogurt
1 frozen banana

4 dates, pitted
¼ cup almond butter

1. In a blender, combine the milk, yogurt, banana, dates, and almond butter. Blend until smooth.
2. Freeze leftovers in ice-pop molds for up to 3 months.

Tip: Add a handful of frozen chopped spinach to this smoothie for extra veggie power. It will change the color but only minimally affect flavor.

Extra Cheesy Egg Muffins

Early Introduction

Freezer-Friendly

Gluten-Free

Healthy Fats

Nut-Free

On the Go

Quick and Easy

Protein-packed breakfasts release consistent energy all morning and help bellies stay full longer because proteins and fats are digested at a much slower rate than carbohydrates. These muffins can postpone the question "Can I have a snack?" immediately after mealtime.

Olive oil or unsalted butter, for greasing

4 ounces cheddar cheese, grated (about 1 cup), divided

12 large eggs

4 ounces cream cheese, at room temperature

1 tablespoon unsalted butter, melted

1. Preheat the oven to 350°F. Lightly grease a 12-cup muffin tin with olive oil.
2. Sprinkle a little less than 1 tablespoon of shredded cheese into each muffin cup.
3. Crack the eggs into a large bowl. Add the cream cheese. Using a handheld mixer, slowly blend the eggs and cream cheese together. While blending, slowly add the melted butter.
4. Scoop the egg and cream cheese mixture into the prepared muffin cups, filling each about two-thirds full.
5. Sprinkle a bit of the remaining cheese over the top of each egg muffin.
6. Bake for about 20 minutes, or until the center is set. Let rest for 5 to 10 minutes before removing the egg muffins from the tin.
7. Store in a sealed container in the refrigerator for up to 3 days or freeze for up to 3 months.

Tip: This recipe is a blank canvas for additional veggies or meats to be added: bacon, ham, peppers, spinach, tomatoes, mushrooms—you name it.

Overnight Oatmeal Waffles

MAKES 6 OR 7 (7-INCH ROUND) WAFFLES

Prep time:
5 minutes, plus overnight to soak the oats
Cook time:
15 minutes

Freezer-Friendly

Healthy Fats

Nut-Free

On the Go

Vegetarian

This rich Belgian waffle–inspired recipe is a particular favorite. Soaking the mixture overnight provides the benefits of soaked oats described on page 30 and deepens the flavors. Kefir, a fermented milk drink, is an excellent source of probiotics and can be found in the yogurt aisle or made easily at home. If you don't have kefir on hand, you can swap in plain yogurt.

2 cups old-fashioned
   rolled oats
½ cup whole wheat flour
1 teaspoon baking powder
1 teaspoon baking soda
1 cup plain whole milk kefir
1 cup whole milk

2 large eggs
6 tablespoons (¾ stick)
   unsalted butter, melted,
   plus extra for greasing
   the waffle iron
2 tablespoons maple syrup
2 teaspoons vanilla extract

1. In a large mixing bowl, whisk together the oats, flour, baking powder, and baking soda.
2. Add the kefir, milk, eggs, butter, maple syrup, and vanilla and stir until just combined.
3. Cover the bowl tightly with plastic wrap and refrigerate for at least 8 hours or overnight.
4. Heat a waffle iron. Remove the mixture from the refrigerator and stir. Once the waffle iron has heated, brush melted butter on the surface.
5. Scoop ½ cup of the batter into the waffle iron, close the top, and cook until steaming slows, 1 to 2 minutes. Repeat with the remaining batter.
6. Store leftovers in a sealed container in the refrigerator for up to 3 days or freeze for up to 3 months.

Creamy Pumpkin Custard

SERVES 8

Prep time:
5 minutes

Cook time
40 minutes

Early Introduction

Freezer-Friendly

Healthy Fats

Iron-Rich

On the Go

Vegetarian

Change up your breakfast with this pumpkin-pie-inspired treat. This recipe feeds a crowd; whip up a batch early in the week and enjoy leftovers on busy mornings. This recipe is high in healthy fats and protein, ensuring that you and your little one will be full until that midmorning snack.

½ cup chopped pecans
½ cup old-fashioned rolled oats
1 tablespoon coarse sugar, such as turbinado
1 teaspoon ground cinnamon
¼ cup unsalted butter, cubed, plus more for greasing

1 (13½-ounce) can full-fat coconut milk
1 (15-ounce) can pumpkin puree
4 large eggs
10 dates, pitted
¼ cup maple syrup
1 teaspoon vanilla extract

1. Preheat the oven to 350°F. Grease a 9-by-13-inch baking dish with butter.
2. In a blender or food processor, combine the pecans, oats, sugar, and cinnamon. Pulse until crumbly. Add the butter and pulse until the texture resembles small peas. Scoop the mixture from the blender into a small bowl and set aside.
3. Without cleaning the blender, combine the coconut milk, pumpkin, eggs, dates, maple syrup, and vanilla in the blender. Blend until smooth and creamy.
4. Spread the custard filling into the prepared baking dish and sprinkle the oat crumble evenly on top.
5. Bake until the custard is set in the middle, about 40 minutes.
6. Store leftovers in a sealed container in the refrigerator for up to 3 days or freeze for up to 3 months.

Simple Scratch Biscuits

MAKES 12 (2-INCH) BISCUITS

Prep time:
10 minutes

Cook time:
15 minutes

Freezer-Friendly

Nut-Free

On the Go

Quick and Easy

Vegetarian

These biscuits are so versatile. Serve them warm with butter, molasses, or jelly. Or serve them alongside Chunky Split Pea Soup (page 52), smothered in gravy, or as the bread for an egg sandwich. Excited? Ready. Set. Bake.

2 cups unbleached all-purpose flour, plus more for dusting
1 tablespoon baking powder
1 tablespoon sugar
1 teaspoon salt

8 tablespoons (1 stick) very cold unsalted butter, divided
¾ cup whole milk, chilled

1. Preheat the oven to 425°F. Line a rimmed baking sheet with parchment or a silicone baking mat.
2. In a large bowl, gently combine the flour with the baking powder, sugar, and salt.
3. Place the box grater on a cutting board and quickly grate 6 tablespoons (¾ stick) of butter; set aside the remaining (ungrated) 2 tablespoons of butter.
4. Scoop the grated butter into the flour bowl, then with 2 forks, push the butter down and away, "cutting" it into the flour until the mixture resembles coarse crumbs and no longer has patches of dry flour.
5. Add the cold milk and, using a wooden spoon, gently mix it into the dough. Be careful not to overmix; the dough should remain sticky.

6. Sprinkle flour onto a clean surface and put a light dusting of flour on your clean hands. Transfer the dough to the floured work surface and gently shape the dough into a ball. Roll the dough ball through the flour, covering all sides, then with the heel of your hands, press the dough down flat. Fold the dough in half, back on top of itself, turn it 90 degrees, then fold the dough in half again, rotate it 90 degrees, press it down flat, then fold again. Repeat this five or six times.

7. With your hands, pat the dough out flat until it's about 1 inch thick, then lightly dust a biscuit cutter or the outer ring of a mason jar lid.

8. Keeping the cuts close, press the biscuit cutter straight down in the dough, give it a wiggle, and transfer the biscuit onto the prepared baking sheet, placing the biscuits side by side so the edges just touch. This will help with the rising.

9. Keep cutting biscuits, then refold and reflatten the dough, until all the dough has been used.

10. Bake for 12 to 14 minutes, or until the tops begin to turn golden.

11. Melt the remaining 2 tablespoons of butter and brush it over the top of the hot biscuits. Serve warm.

12. Store leftovers in a sealed container at room temperature for 3 days, refrigerate for up to 1 week, or freeze for up to 3 months.

Tip: The colder the butter, the better! If you remember, stick the butter in the freezer for 15 to 20 minutes before starting—or even up to an hour. This will keep the grating mess to a minimum, help the biscuits rise to their fullest potential, and fill each bite with a tiny drop of buttery goodness.

Broccoli Quiche with Oat Crust

SERVES 6

Prep time:
5 minutes

Cook time:
45 minutes

Healthy Fats

Nut-Free

Vegetarian

Quiche is one of our favorite last-minute meal ideas for both breakfast and dinner for a few reasons. For one thing, we usually have all of the ingredients on hand, but also quiche is a delicious way to get in a serving of veggies. Although this recipe uses broccoli, you can use 2 cups of whatever mix-ins you have available; for example, peppers and sausage, asparagus and onions, zucchini and tomato. It is even delicious with no crust at all!

1¼ cups old-fashioned
    rolled oats
¼ teaspoon salt
4 tablespoons (½ stick) cold
    unsalted butter, cubed
¼ cup cold water
6 large eggs

1 cup whole milk
2 cups chopped broccoli
½ teaspoon freshly
    ground black pepper
1 cup shredded cheddar
    cheese (about 4 ounces)

1. Preheat the oven to 350°F.
2. Put the oats in a blender or food processor and blend until a fine flour forms.
3. In a medium bowl, combine the oat flour and salt. With a fork or your fingers, cut the butter into the flour and salt until the mixture resembles crumbly sand. Stir in the cold water. Use your clean hands to work the dough together, then form it into a ball.
4. Press the dough evenly into the sides and bottom of a 9-inch pie pan, then place it in the refrigerator until ready to use (this keeps the butter from softening).

5. In a medium bowl, combine the eggs and milk and whisk until smooth. Add in the broccoli and pepper and whisk again. Pour the egg mixture into the prepared crust and top with the shredded cheese.
6. Bake for 40 to 45 minutes, or until the quiche is completely set in the center.
7. Store leftovers in a sealed container in the refrigerator for up to 3 days.

Tip: Frozen broccoli also works well in this recipe. Simply chop it while frozen and stir it into the eggs.

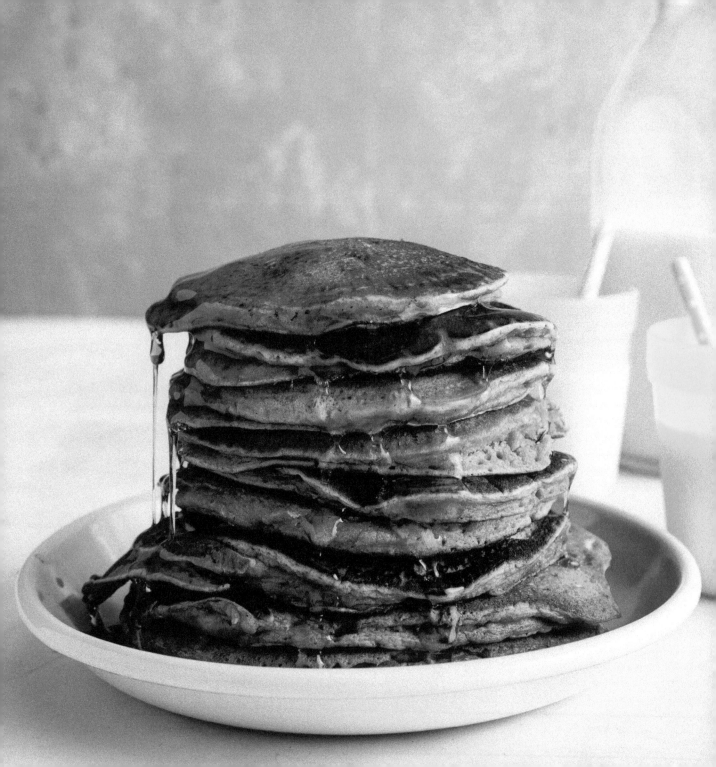

Hot Pink Pancakes

MAKES 8 TO 10 (3- TO 4-INCH) PANCAKES

Prep time:
10 minutes

Cook time:
15 minutes

Freezer-Friendly

Nut-Free

On the Go

Quick and Easy

Vegetarian

We know some toddlers who are pretty thrilled about the idea of hot pink pancakes. And when we say hot pink, we mean it—these pancakes are vivid. Although we often recommend introducing veggies in their whole form, adding a beet to a classic, fluffy pancake recipe is a great way to introduce a new, complex flavor in a food that is familiar to many little ones. Beets are a great way to add bright color to smoothies as well.

1 beet, boiled, peeled, and cooled, or ¼ cup canned beets, drained and rinsed

1 cup whole milk

1 large egg

1 tablespoon coconut oil, at room temperature, plus more for greasing

2 tablespoons maple syrup

1 teaspoon vanilla extract

1 cup unbleached all-purpose flour

1 teaspoon baking powder

1 teaspoon baking soda

¼ teaspoon salt

1. In a blender, combine the beets with the milk and blend until smooth (and bright pink!).
2. Add the egg, coconut oil, maple syrup, and vanilla and blend until well combined.
3. Add the flour, baking powder, baking soda, and salt and pulse until just combined.

CONTINUED

4. Heat a large cast-iron skillet over medium heat. Grease the skillet with coconut oil. Pour about ¼ cup pancake batter into the skillet for each pancake and cook for 3 to 4 minutes, or until bubbles begin to form on the surface. Flip and cook for about 1 minute more. Repeat with the remaining batter (if your skillet is large enough, you can cook more than one pancake at a time; just space them so they don't run together).

5. Store leftovers in a sealed container in the refrigerator for up to 3 days or freeze for up to 3 months.

Tip: For frozen pancakes and waffles that won't stick together, lay cooked cakes in a flat layer on a baking sheet and freeze until solid. Once frozen, pop them off the baking sheet and into a freezer bag or other sealed container. Reheat from frozen in the toaster before serving.

G'ma Hill's Cornbread with Homemade Butter

SERVES 8

Prep time:
25 minutes

Cook time:
25 minutes

Nut-Free

Vegetarian

A good chunk of cornbread can take any meal from good to great. Passed down from several generations in the Gipson family and developed when all recipes used whole foods, this old-fashioned scratch batter has stood the test of time. We thought this crispy cornbread would pair perfectly with a big ol' dollop of pearly homemade butter. You can even recycle the fresh-made buttermilk from the homemade butter into the cornbread recipe!

For the homemade butter

2 cups heavy cream (at least 36% butterfat), divided

2 cups ice water
1 teaspoon salt (optional)

For the cornbread

1 cup white cornmeal
2 tablespoons unbleached all-purpose flour
½ teaspoon baking soda
1 teaspoon baking powder
1 teaspoon salt
2 tablespoons sugar

1 cup buttermilk (can be combined with extracted buttermilk from the homemade butter recipe)
1 large egg
2 tablespoons homemade butter

CONTINUED

1. **To make the homemade butter:** Pour 2 cups of heavy cream into the bowl of a stand mixer fitted with the wire whisk attachment or into a large bowl if you will use a handheld mixer. Begin whipping the cream on low speed (expect some splashing), then increase the speed to medium. Watch carefully during the next 5 to 10 minutes; first, the cream will begin to thicken and transform into soft whipped cream, then soft peaks will break, liquid will begin to separate, and you'll see butter begin to cling to the beater wires.

2. Once the butter has solidified, pour the resulting buttermilk into a separate container for storage, or you can use it for the cornbread recipe.

3. Scoop the solid butter into a bowl and rinse it by pouring ice water over it and pressing out the remaining buttermilk with a small spatula or a spoon.

4. Pour off the water and repeat the process. Keep rinsing and squishing the butter until the water runs clear. Then, stir in the salt (if using), thoroughly working it through the butter.

5. Transfer the butter to a container with a tight-fitting lid and store in the refrigerator for up to 3 weeks.

6. **To make the cornbread:** Preheat the oven to 425°F.
7. In a large bowl, combine the cornmeal, flour, baking soda, baking powder, salt, and sugar.
8. Add the buttermilk and egg and mix well.
9. On the stovetop, heat the 2 tablespoons butter in a large cast-iron skillet over medium heat. When the butter has melted and is beginning to sizzle, swirl the skillet around to coat the bottom and sides with butter.
10. Pour the batter into the hot skillet. Let sizzle for about 30 seconds. Remove from the burner and bake in the oven for about 15 to 20 minutes, or until golden brown.
11. Working quickly, remove the skillet from the oven. Using a spatula, flip the entire cornbread over in the skillet and immediately place it back into the oven to bake for an additional 5 minutes. Serve warm with the homemade butter.

Tip: If you don't have buttermilk on hand for the cornbread, here is a quick DIY conversion: 1 tablespoon white vinegar + enough milk to measure 1 cup = 1 cup buttermilk. Lemon juice instead of vinegar works, too! Just let the mixture sit for about 5 minutes to thicken. And if you're short on time, you can skip making the butter altogether and use store-bought.

Tropical Breakfast Cookie Bites

MAKES ABOUT 24 COOKIES

Prep time:
15 minutes

Cook time:
15 minutes

Freezer-Friendly

Healthy Fats

On the Go

Quick and Easy

Vegetarian

These breakfast treats are loaded with tasty tropical flavors like banana, pineapple, and coconut along with the warm spices ginger and cinnamon. Oat-based cookies like these are a great alternative to packaged bars for babies on the go.

2 cups quick-cooking oats
1 cup unbleached
    all-purpose flour
¼ cup ground flaxseed
1 teaspoon baking powder
½ teaspoon ground cinnamon
½ teaspoon ground ginger
¼ teaspoon salt
½ cup unsweetened
    shredded coconut

½ cup finely chopped
    pecans or walnuts
¼ cup dried pineapple,
    finely chopped
¼ cup mini chocolate
    chips (optional)
2 ripe bananas
3 tablespoons maple syrup
4 tablespoons (½ stick)
    unsalted butter, melted
1 large egg

1. Preheat the oven to 350°F. Line 2 rimmed baking sheets with parchment paper.
2. In a large bowl, whisk together the oats, flour, flaxseed, baking powder, cinnamon, ginger, salt, coconut, pecans, pineapple, and chocolate chips (if using).
3. In a medium mixing bowl, mash the bananas, then stir in the maple syrup, melted butter, and egg until combined.
4. Pour the wet ingredients into the dry ingredients and stir until combined.

5. Scoop 1½ to 2 tablespoons of the dough onto the prepared baking sheets about 2 inches apart, pressing them down with a fork to flatten.
6. Bake for 15 minutes, or until golden brown.
7. Store leftovers in a sealed container at room temperature for up to 3 days, refrigerate for up to 1 week, or freeze for up to 3 months.

Tip: These freeze well both before and after baking. To freeze the dough, follow the recipe through step 5 and then place the baking sheets in the freezer until the raw dough is frozen solid. Pop the frozen dough balls into a freezer-safe container and store for up to 3 months. Bake from frozen following the instructions, increasing baking time by about 3 minutes.

Rose Velvet First Birthday Cake

**MAKES
1 (6-INCH)
TRIPLE LAYER
CAKE OR
1 (8-INCH)
DOUBLE
LAYER CAKE**

Prep time:
30 minutes,
plus
20 minutes
to cool for
each cake

Cook time:
30 minutes for
each cake

Vegetarian

This recipe is named in honor of Ellen's newest niece, Clara Rose, inspired and meticulously tested with her cake-connoisseur sister, co-owner of the Cake Mom & Co. Free of artificial food coloring, the subtle rose hue of this cake comes from bright red beets. The finished product is generously layered with rich homemade whipped cream.

For the cake

Nonstick cooking spray,
    for greasing
1 (15-ounce) can
    beets, drained, with
    juice reserved
4 tablespoons (½ stick)
    unsalted butter, at room
    temperature, plus more
    for greasing
¾ cup buttermilk

¼ cup sugar
¼ cup maple syrup
2 large eggs
1 teaspoon vanilla extract
2 teaspoons cocoa powder
½ teaspoon salt
2½ cups unbleached
    cake flour
1 tablespoon white vinegar
1 teaspoon baking soda

For the whipped cream

2 cups heavy
    (whipping) cream

1 teaspoon vanilla extract

1. **To make the cake:** Preheat the oven to 350°F.
2. Trace the bottom circumference of the cake pans on parchment paper, then cut out either three 6-inch circles or two 8-inch circles. Grease the bottom of the pans with butter and secure the parchment rounds in the bottom of the pan. Coat the paper and sides of the pan with cooking spray.

3. In a blender, puree the drained beets until liquefied. Measure out ¾ cup of the beet puree. Set it aside in a small bowl.

4. Then, in another small bowl, mix together the buttermilk with ¼ cup of the reserved beet juice (you will need an additional ¼ cup beet juice in step 5).

5. Put the butter, sugar, and maple syrup in a large bowl. Using an electric mixer or a stand mixer, beat until creamy. Add the eggs, one at a time, beating well after each addition. Gently mix in another ¼ cup of reserved beet juice, ¾ cup of beet puree, and the vanilla.

6. Add the cocoa and salt, then alternately mix in the flour and buttermilk/beet mixture.

7. Gently fold in the vinegar and baking soda, making sure they are thoroughly incorporated.

8. Evenly divide and pour the batter into the prepared pans. Bake for 25 to 30 minutes, until the cakes begin to pull away from the sides of the pans or a toothpick inserted in the center comes out clean.

9. Set the pans on a wire rack to cool for 10 to 20 minutes. Turn the cakes out of the pans directly onto the wire rack and let them cool completely.

10. **To make the whipped cream:** In a large mixing bowl, whip the cream on high speed for 3 to 5 minutes, or until stiff peaks form. (Do not overbeat.) Gently fold in the vanilla. Store the whipped cream in a covered container in the refrigerator until ready to spread between the layers and over the top of the completely cooled cakes.

Tip: To give a pink hue to the whipped cream, add 2 to 3 teaspoons of the reserved beet juice.

Cranberry Pistachio Bars

MAKES 16 TO 18 (1-BY-3-INCH) BARS

Prep time:
5 minutes, plus 15 minutes to chill and set

Cook time:
10 minutes

Freezer-Friendly

On the Go

Quick and Easy

Vegetarian

Making homemade granola bars seems like a big task, but it can be very simple. Think of this recipe as a template for delicious granola bars that you can modify to your preferences. Pick a dried fruit and nut variety, then mix and match. We chose deep red cranberries and cool green pistachios, appealing to the eyes and belly.

2 cups old-fashioned rolled oats

1 cup shelled, unsalted pistachios, finely chopped

1 cup unsweetened dried cranberries

1 tablespoon chia seeds

4 tablespoons (½ stick) unsalted butter

¼ cup maple syrup

⅓ cup packed dark brown sugar

½ teaspoon vanilla extract

1. Line a 9-by-13-inch baking pan with parchment paper.
2. In a large bowl, mix together the oats, pistachios, cranberries, and chia seeds.
3. In a small saucepan, over medium heat, cook the butter, maple syrup, and brown sugar until it starts to bubble, about 5 minutes. Reduce the heat to low and continue to cook at a low boil for about 2 minutes. Remove from the heat, add the vanilla, and stir.
4. Pour the syrup mixture over the dry ingredients and mix well until all the dry ingredients are moistened.

5. Press the mixture evenly into the prepared pan with a spoon or clean hands.
6. Set in the refrigerator to cool for about 15 minutes. Cut into rectangles about 1 by 3 inches and serve.
7. Store leftovers in a sealed container at room temperature for 3 days, refrigerate for up to 1 week, or freeze for up to 3 months.

Tip: These chewy granola bars are great for a breakfast or snack on the go. We don't recommend unsafe habits, like eating in the car seat or while physically walking or moving, but as mobility increases, so do busy schedules and the necessity for portable food. To keep messes contained throughout the home, designate preapproved eating locations away from the family table, like a picnic blanket, toddler snack table, or porch step.

White Bean–Ranch Hummus and Veggies

MAKES 1½ CUPS HUMMUS

Prep time: 10 minutes

Freezer-Friendly

Gluten-Free

Healthy Fats

Iron-Rich

No-Cook

Nut-Free

On the Go

Quick and Easy

Vegetarian

Beans are an amazing food for babies, and really for people of all ages. They're energy dense, high fiber, and a good iron source as well as a cost-effective protein that adapts to many recipes. When in doubt, add a can of beans. Although traditional hummus is made with tahini (paste made of sesame seeds) and chickpeas (garbanzo beans), we've made a few convenience and cost tweaks to deliver a whole new taste. Building our own ranch spice blend to pair with mild white beans gives this veggie dip a punch of flavor.

1 (15-ounce) can low-sodium great northern beans, drained and rinsed
2 tablespoons water
2 tablespoons olive oil
1 tablespoon fresh lemon juice
1 teaspoon garlic powder
2 teaspoons onion flakes
2 teaspoons dried parsley
1 teaspoon dried dill

½ teaspoon freshly ground black pepper
½ teaspoon freeze-dried chives
1 tablespoon dry buttermilk powder
1 teaspoon salt (optional)
1 cup sliced vegetables, such as celery, carrots, bell peppers, zucchini, or jicama

1. In a blender, combine the beans, water, olive oil, lemon juice, garlic powder, onion flakes, parsley, dill, black pepper, chives, buttermilk powder, and salt (if using). Blend until smooth. Scrape down the sides and blend again, if necessary.
2. Serve with the sliced veggies. Store the hummus in a sealed container in the refrigerator for up to 7 days or freeze for up to 3 months.

Tip: Buttermilk powder can be found in the baking aisle of the grocery store.

Irresistible Kale Chips

**MAKES
1½ CUPS**

Prep time:
5 minutes

Cook time:
15 minutes

Gluten-Free

Healthy Fats

Iron-Rich

Nut-Free

Quick and Easy

Vegan

A simple, salty whole food snack in 15 minutes? Kale, yeah! Before 2007, these dark greens were merely a garnish served next to your steak frites and presumed inedible, but by 2012, kale had earned itself a 400 percent increase on restaurant menus. Today kale is a staple for many households and still a nutrient powerhouse, so we are proud to include these crispy snackin' chips as an ol' faithful adult- and kid-friendly recipe. For even quicker prep, use prewashed and chopped bagged kale.

1 bunch kale, rinsed and well dried (about 7 ounces or 3 cups prepped and torn)

1 tablespoon olive oil
Sea salt

1. Preheat the oven to 350°F. Line a rimmed baking sheet with parchment paper.
2. Carefully remove the kale leaves from their stems and tear or cut the leaves into small "chips," roughly 2-inch pieces.
3. Lay the kale pieces on the prepared baking sheet and drizzle with the olive oil, toss with a wooden spoon, arrange them in a single layer, and sprinkle with sea salt.
4. Bake for 12 to 15 minutes, or until the edges are beginning to brown and they are crisp.
5. Store cooled leftovers in a sealed container at room temperature. They are best if eaten the day they're made.

Tip: These kale chips are a blank canvas for flavor. Experiment with your own favorite spice combinations, like seasoned salt, a Cajun blend, curry and turmeric, or sweet maple.

Turkey and Avocado Roll-Up

SERVES 1

Prep time:
5 minutes

Dairy-Free

Healthy Fats

Iron-Rich

No-Cook

Nut-Free

On the Go

Quick and Easy

Although super simple, this whole food combo is too great of a snack or lunch idea not to share. When it comes to choosing deli meat, look for whole cuts that are free of nitrates, and aim to include deli meat in your child's diet only occasionally. These little bites are full of healthy fats and protein to keep little tummies full. It's a quick, real-food response to that famous question, "Mom, can I have a snack?"

½ avocado, sliced into strips

2 ounces thinly sliced deli turkey

Wrap each avocado strip with a slice of turkey, cutting the turkey slices to fit, if needed. Serve immediately or place in a sealed container and use within 2 days.

Tip: Whip up a batch of Taco Dip (page 81) for dipping.

Crispy Herbed Snackin' Beans

MAKES 3¼ CUPS

Prep time:
10 minutes

Cook time:
45 minutes

Dairy-Free

Gluten-Free

Healthy Fats

Iron-Rich

Nut-Free

On the Go

Vegan

Move over Goldfish, there's a new snack in town. These crispy beans are as addicting as those famous snack crackers, but way more satisfying. Packed with protein and fiber, this simple recipe transforms white beans into light and crispy bites that you don't want to stop eating.

2 (15-ounce) cans low-sodium cannellini or great northern beans, drained and rinsed

¼ cup olive oil

½ teaspoon garlic powder

1 tablespoon chopped fresh thyme, or 1 teaspoon dried thyme

1 tablespoon chopped fresh oregano, or 1 teaspoon dried oregano

¼ teaspoon salt

1. Preheat the oven to 425°F.
2. Spread the drained beans on a clean dish towel or paper towels for about 5 minutes to remove any excess moisture.
3. In a large mixing bowl, drizzle the beans with the olive oil and sprinkle with the garlic powder, thyme, oregano, and salt. Toss to coat and spread in a single layer on a rimmed baking sheet.
4. Bake for 45 minutes, stirring at least once, until browned and crispy.
5. Store leftovers in a sealed container in the refrigerator for up to 1 week.

Tip: This recipe is super versatile. Try different flavor combinations or even dry ranch seasoning mix.

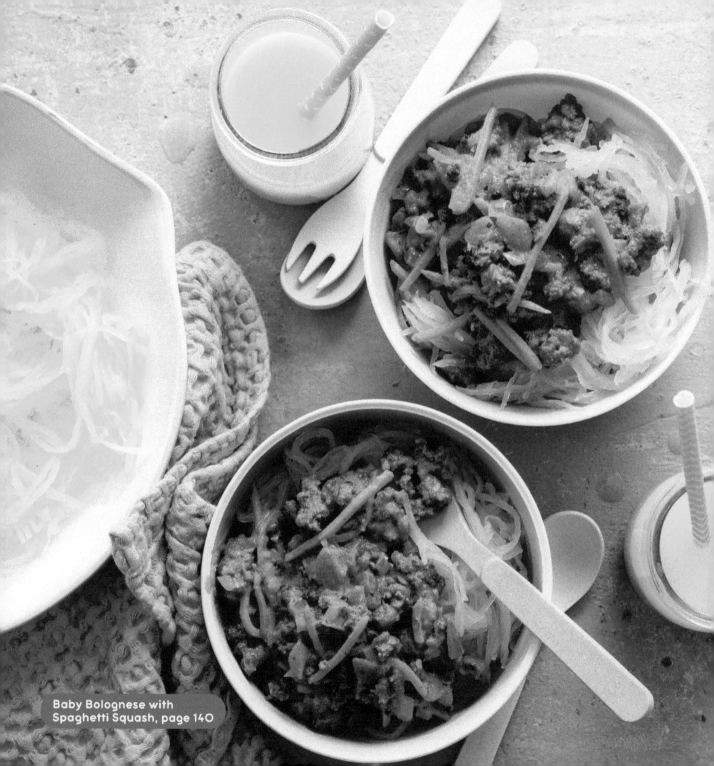

Baby Bolognese with
Spaghetti Squash, page 140

CHAPTER 6
Family Lunches and Dinners
(12 Months and Up)

Now that you have a 1-year-old, mealtimes may be a little less peaceful and a little more active. You may even notice some selective eating behaviors popping up. Now is the time to really stick to offering a wide variety of nutrient-packed foods, even if they are sometimes rejected. The role of our little ones is to decide what or even if they will eat, while we as caregivers continue to offer nutrient-packed foods (and strive not to give in).

The recipes in this chapter continue to keep key nutrients and allergen introduction in mind, while presenting more of an emphasis on eating the same meals together as a family. Babies and toddlers learn so much from parents and older siblings at the table. Portion sizes vary widely for babies around this age. Little ones can be overwhelmed easily by a large plate of food, so it is always a good bet to start small, especially when introducing new foods, then offer more only as needed.

One-Pan Southwest Quinoa

SERVES 4

Prep time:
5 minutes

Cook time:
35 minutes

Gluten-Free

Iron-Rich

Nut-Free

On the Go

Vegetarian

A go-to dish for busy nights, this Mexican-inspired dish comes together quickly. Sautéing the dry quinoa first lends a deep toasty flavor that lingers even as it soaks up all the seasonings. Serve this dish on its own or as the base for a taco bowl topped with shredded pork or chicken.

3 tablespoons olive oil
1 cup quinoa, rinsed
   and drained
1 teaspoon ground cumin
1 onion, finely chopped
1 garlic clove, minced
1 (15-ounce) can low-
   sodium black beans,
   drained and rinsed

1 cup frozen corn
1 (14½-ounce) can diced
   tomatoes, no salt added
1½ cups water
¼ teaspoon sea salt
Sliced avocado and
   plain whole milk
   yogurt, for serving

1. In a large cast-iron skillet, heat the oil over medium heat. Add the quinoa and sauté until fragrant and lightly browned, about 10 minutes. Stir in the cumin, onion, and garlic and sauté for about 5 minutes, or until the onion is translucent.
2. Add the beans, corn, tomatoes, water, and salt.
3. Bring to a boil, then cover and reduce the heat to medium-low. Simmer for 20 minutes, or until all of the liquid is absorbed and the quinoa is fluffy. Serve with sliced avocado and yogurt.
4. Store leftovers in a sealed container in the refrigerator for up to 3 days.

Ricotta Gnocchi with Spinach and Butter Thyme Sauce

Early Introduction

Healthy Fats

Iron-Rich

Nut-Free

Vegetarian

A few months into the solid food journey, we often hear from parents that they have run out of ideas for what to try next. Maybe baby has already developed a few favorites, so it becomes easy to stick to what they already know. Enter gnocchi, soft little dumplings that are calorically dense, accepted by picky eaters, and a great vehicle for flavor-packed sauces.

1 (15-ounce) container whole milk ricotta cheese

2 eggs, lightly beaten

1¼ cups grated Parmesan cheese

¾ to 1 cup unbleached all-purpose flour, divided

4 tablespoons (½ stick) butter

1 garlic clove, minced

3 tablespoons fresh thyme leaves, or 1½ teaspoons dried thyme

2 cups spinach, sliced into thin ribbons

1. Fill a large stockpot two-thirds full with water and bring the water to a rolling boil over medium-high heat.
2. While the water is heating, combine the ricotta cheese, eggs, Parmesan, and ¾ cup of flour in a large mixing bowl. Add more flour, 1 tablespoon at a time, until a sticky dough forms (you may need to bring the dough together with your clean hands).

3. Test the dough by rolling about 1 tablespoon into a ball and sliding it into the boiling water. If the dough ball loses its shape, add more flour to the dough, 1 tablespoon at a time, then retest.

4. In a medium skillet, melt the butter over medium heat and cook until golden brown with light brown flecks and a nutty aroma develops, about 3 minutes. Add the garlic and thyme and cook for 3 minutes, or until fragrant. Turn off the heat, but keep the skillet warm.

5. While the butter is browning, form the dough into dumplings: Press the dough into a 1- to 2-inch-thick rectangle and cut it into small 1-inch squares using a pastry cutter or knife.

6. Drop the dumplings into the boiling water. To avoid overcrowding the pot, boil 7 to 10 dumplings at a time. When the gnocchi float to the surface, after 2 to 3 minutes, they are done. Remove the gnocchi with a slotted spoon, draining as much water as possible, and transfer them to the warm skillet with the browned butter and thyme.

7. Stir to coat the gnocchi with the butter sauce. Add the shredded spinach and toss it in the butter sauce before serving.

8. Store leftovers in a sealed container in the refrigerator for up to 3 days.

Tip: This gnocchi pairs well with many different kinds of sauce, such as Bolognese (see page 140) or simply a low-sodium jarred marinara topped with Parmesan.

Quick Chickpea Coconut Curry

SERVES 4

Prep time:
5 minutes

Cook time:
30 minutes

Dairy-Free

Gluten-Free

Healthy Fats

Iron-Rich

Vegan

Babies' palates have unlimited potential. Babies from all over the world grow up loving flavors, spices, and textures unique to their cultures, so we know that babies can find enjoyment and sustenance from a wide range of first foods. This curry is a great example.

1 tablespoon coconut oil

1 small onion, chopped

1 red or yellow bell pepper, chopped

2 cups chopped fresh spinach

3 garlic cloves, minced

½ teaspoon ground ginger, or 1 tablespoon chopped fresh ginger

1 tablespoon curry powder

¼ teaspoon sea salt

2 (15-ounce) cans low-sodium chickpeas, drained and rinsed

1 (13½-ounce) can full-fat coconut milk

2 tablespoons freshly squeezed lemon or lime juice

¼ cup chopped fresh basil, for topping

1. In a large skillet, melt the coconut oil over medium heat. Add the onion, bell pepper, spinach, and garlic and sauté for 7 to 10 minutes, or until soft. Add the ginger, curry powder, and salt and continue to cook, stirring frequently, for 2 to 3 minutes, or until fragrant and well combined.
2. Add the chickpeas and the coconut milk and allow to simmer, covered, for 15 minutes. Stir in the lemon juice, top with basil, and serve.
3. Store leftovers in a sealed container in the refrigerator for up to 3 days.

Tip: Serve this curry with Coconut Rice (page 128) and a warm pita or naan. Any sturdy green like bok choy or kale can be used in place of the spinach.

Nourishing Lentil Stew

**SERVES
4 TO 6**

Prep time:
15 minutes

Cook time:
1 hour
20 minutes

Dairy-Free

Freezer-Friendly

Iron-Rich

Nut-Free

Vegan

This comforting soup features hearty lentils along with wholesome vegetables. Serving soup to babies and toddlers can be a messy business, but practice makes perfect. Although you can certainly serve this soup with a spoon, also try offering chunks of crusty bread for dipping.

2 tablespoons olive oil

1 onion, chopped

3 garlic cloves, minced

4 carrots, sliced

1 large sweet potato,
peeled and chopped

3 large celery stalks, sliced

7 cups low-sodium vegetable
broth or water, divided

1½ cups lentils, rinsed

1 (28-ounce) can diced
tomatoes, no salt added

2 tablespoons tomato paste

1 teaspoon dried rosemary

1 bay leaf

½ teaspoon sea salt

1. In a large stockpot or Dutch oven, heat the oil over medium heat. Add the onion and garlic and cook until fragrant, 3 to 5 minutes. Add the carrots, sweet potato, and celery and cook for 10 to 15 minutes more, or until the vegetables brown slightly on the bottom.

2. Pour in about 1 cup of broth and use a wooden spoon to deglaze the pot by scraping up the brown bits on the bottom of the pot. Add the remaining broth, the lentils, tomatoes, tomato paste, rosemary, bay leaf, and salt and bring to a boil. Reduce the heat to medium-low and simmer, covered, for at least 30 minutes or up to 60 minutes for even deeper flavor. Remove the bay leaf before serving.

3. Store leftovers in a sealed container in the refrigerator for up to 3 days or freeze in a large container or individual portions for up to 3 months.

Simple Roast Chicken

Prep time:
5 minutes, plus
15 minutes to
cool

Cook time:
1 hour

Gluten-Free

Healthy Fats

Iron-Rich

Nut-Free

On the Go

Few things can make a home smell more delicious than a roasting chicken. Though roasting a whole bird seems a little intimidating at first, this simple and delicious recipe goes from oven to table without much fuss. You will likely have some leftover chicken, which is great to have on hand as a high-quality protein option for quick toddler lunches. Remove it from the bone-in strips or bite-size pieces before serving, or let baby have a leg to themselves.

3 tablespoons olive oil, divided

1 (4- to 5-pound) whole chicken

1 teaspoon dried thyme

½ teaspoon dried rosemary

1 teaspoon sea salt

½ teaspoon freshly ground black pepper

1 lemon, sliced into rounds

3 thyme sprigs

2 rosemary sprigs

3 garlic cloves, smashed

1 onion, roughly chopped

1. Preheat the oven to 450°F.
2. Drizzle 1 tablespoon of olive oil in a large cast-iron skillet or Dutch oven. Place the chicken in the skillet and rub the remaining 2 tablespoons of olive oil over the entire bird.
3. Season the chicken with the dried thyme, dried rosemary, salt, and pepper. Arrange the lemon slices, thyme sprigs, and rosemary sprigs on top of the chicken. Stuff the chicken with the garlic and onion.

4. Roast for 45 minutes, then remove the chicken from the oven and spoon the juices over the chicken. Return it to the oven and roast for 10 to 15 minutes more, or until the internal temperature of the thickest part of the breast reaches 165°F.
5. Allow the chicken to cool for 10 to 15 minutes, then slice and serve.
6. Store leftovers in a sealed container in the refrigerator for up to 3 days.

Tip: For a deeper flavor, season the chicken with the olive oil, dried thyme, dried rosemary, salt, and pepper the night before cooking. Keep it in the refrigerator until ready to roast (mine goes, covered, in the Dutch oven that it gets cooked in).

Everything Fried Rice

SERVES 4

Prep time:
10 minutes

Cook time:
20 minutes

Early Introduction

Iron-Rich

Nut-Free

Quick and Easy

Vegetarian

Who doesn't love a one-pan meal? In this version of fried rice, everything goes! Feel free to make it your own. Recipes like this are great for utilizing leftovers: extra grilled zucchini, roasted cauliflower, fresh pineapple, sliced ham, chopped peanuts, sautéed mushrooms, edamame, grilled shrimp—throw it in! Exposing children to familiar foods in different formats and new presentations is a simple way to keep things exciting.

4 tablespoons (½ stick) unsalted butter, divided
1 head broccoli, cut into florets
2 large carrots, grated
1 tablespoon minced garlic
½ cup frozen green peas

½ cup diced onion
3 eggs
3 cups cooked brown rice
⅓ cup low-sodium soy sauce
Sea salt
Freshly ground black pepper

1. In a large cast-iron skillet over medium-high heat, melt 1 tablespoon of butter. Add the broccoli and carrots and sauté for about 5 minutes, or until softened. Add 1 tablespoon of butter, as well as the garlic, green peas, and onion. Cook another 5 minutes, or until all of the vegetables are tender and slightly browned. Transfer to a medium bowl.
2. In a small bowl, whisk the eggs. In the same cast-iron skillet, melt another tablespoon of butter over medium-high heat. Pour the eggs into the skillet. Cook the eggs until almost firm on one side, about 90 seconds. Using a spatula, flip the eggs. Cook on the other side for 30 to 45 seconds, or until cooked through. Transfer the eggs to a cutting board and chop them into small pieces.

3. In the same cast-iron skillet, melt the remaining tablespoon of butter over medium-high heat and cook until it begins to sizzle. Add the rice and smooth it flat with a spatula to fill the entire pan. Fry undisturbed for 1 to 2 minutes, then stir. Fry, stirring occasionally, for 2 to 3 minutes more or until heated through.

4. Add the cooked veggies and chopped egg to the rice in the skillet. Pour in the soy sauce and season with salt and pepper.

5. Store leftovers in a sealed container in the refrigerator for up to 3 days.

Tip: If you are using leftovers in this recipe, decrease the cook time in step 1. You will need to heat the leftovers only until they are warm.

Crispy Black Bean Skillet Tacos

**MAKES
8 TACOS**

Prep time:
10 minutes

Cook time:
20 minutes

Gluten-Free

Healthy Fats

Iron-Rich

Nut-Free

On the Go

Quick and Easy

Vegetarian

This meal is perfect for those nights when you need dinner to come together as quickly as possible. It's also a classic kid favorite: crispy taco shells enveloping gooey cheese and cozy black beans. Corn tortillas can be tricky to work with, but warming them increases pliability.

3 to 4 tablespoons
    olive oil, divided
2 cups cooked or canned
    low-sodium black beans,
    drained and rinsed
½ cup minced red onion
1 teaspoon ground cumin

1 teaspoon paprika
8 (6-inch) corn tortillas
2 cups grated cheddar cheese
    (about 8 ounces), divided
Plain whole milk yogurt,
    salsa, and sliced
    avocado, for serving

1. In a large cast-iron skillet, heat 1 tablespoon of olive oil over medium heat.
2. While the oil is heating, in a medium bowl, combine the beans, red onion, cumin, and paprika and mash them together with a fork.
3. Place 2 or 3 corn tortillas flat in the skillet and allow them to heat for about 2 minutes until they are soft and pliable. Top each with ¼ cup of bean mixture and 2 tablespoons of cheese. Gently fold the tortilla over and press it down with a spatula. If the tortilla doesn't stay folded, place the bottom of a clean ceramic bowl on top of it to press it down. Heat for about 3 minutes on each side.

4. Repeat with the remaining ingredients, adding an additional tablespoon of oil before cooking a new round of tacos and working quickly to avoid overheating the oil.
5. Allow the tacos to cool slightly, then serve with yogurt, salsa, and avocado.
6. Store leftover assembled tacos in a sealed container in the refrigerator for up to 3 days.

Tip: To make corn tortillas easier to work with, instead of heating them for 2 minutes in a skillet (as in step 3), you can wrap a stack of tortillas in a damp dish towel and microwave them for 20 seconds prior to using.

Sesame Salmon and Green Beans

SERVES 4

Prep time:
5 minutes

Cook time:
10 minutes

Dairy-Free

Early Introduction

Gluten-Free

Nut-Free

Quick and Easy

Vegetarian

Sesame has emerged as the ninth most common food allergy, shifting the Big 8 to the Big 9. As with all of the major food allergens, early and regular introduction is key for allergy prevention. Sesame oil has a distinct and delicious flavor that is great for stir-frying vegetables, whisking into salad dressings, and marinating meats.

1½ pounds fresh green beans, washed and trimmed

2 tablespoons sesame oil, divided

1 teaspoon minced garlic

2 pounds salmon fillet, skin on

2 tablespoons toasted sesame seeds

Sea salt (optional)

Freshly ground black pepper (optional)

1. Cover the bottom of a medium saucepan with 2 to 3 inches of water and bring it to a simmer over medium heat. Put the green beans into a steamer basket or stainless-steel colander and set it over the simmering water. Steam until the beans have turned bright green, about 2 minutes. Transfer the beans to a colander (if they aren't already in one) and rinse under cold water. Drain well.

2. In a large cast-iron skillet, heat 1 tablespoon of sesame oil over medium-high heat. When it has warmed, swirl the pan to coat the bottom and sides of the pan. Add the garlic and cook for 30 seconds, or until lightly browned. Add the salmon fillet, skin-side down. Cover and cook for 5 minutes, then flip over.

3. Add the remaining tablespoon of sesame oil. Scatter the green beans around the salmon, cover, and cook an additional 5 to 7 minutes, or until the salmon is flaky and the internal temperature reaches 145°F.
4. Sprinkle the sesame seeds over the fish and green beans and season with salt and pepper (if using).
5. Store leftovers in a sealed container in the refrigerator for up to 3 days.

Tip: Skin-on salmon provides extra nutrients and flavor, but depending on your preferences, the skin can either be left in place or removed before eating.

Taco Tuna Salad

SERVES 4

Prep time:
15 minutes

Cook time:
10 minutes

Early Introduction

Healthy Fats

Nut-Free

Quick and Easy

A meal without having to turn on the oven is always a win in our books! Made of staple ingredients that you may not realize you already have, this dish lets you stay outside and watch the sunset with the kids instead of standing over the stove all evening.

For the taco seasoning

1 teaspoon chili powder

1½ teaspoons ground cumin

½ teaspoon paprika

¼ teaspoon sea salt

½ teaspoon garlic powder

¼ teaspoon onion powder

¼ teaspoon dried oregano

¼ teaspoon freshly
   ground black pepper

For the tuna salad

1 tablespoon olive oil

½ cup diced red bell pepper

½ cup diced green bell pepper

½ cup diced onion

1 teaspoon minced garlic

2 (5-ounce) cans tuna,
   drained and flaked

½ cup plain whole milk
   Greek yogurt

¼ cup cooked or canned
   low-sodium black beans,
   drained and rinsed

2 eggs, hard-boiled,
   peeled, and chopped

¼ cup sour cream or whole
   milk yogurt (optional)

1 to 2 tablespoons taco
   seasoning, homemade
   or store-bought

Juice of ½ lime (optional)

1. **To make the taco seasoning:** In a small mason jar or bowl, combine the chili powder, cumin, paprika, salt, garlic and onion powders, oregano, and pepper. Stir or shake to combine.
2. **To make the tuna salad:** In a small saucepan, heat the olive oil over medium-high heat. Add the red and green bell peppers, onion, and garlic and sauté until tender and nicely browned, 5 to 7 minutes. Set aside to cool.
3. In a medium bowl, mix together the tuna, yogurt, beans, hard-boiled eggs, and sour cream (if using). Stir in the taco seasoning until fully incorporated. Add the lime juice (if using).
4. Store in a sealed container in the refrigerator for up to 3 days.

Tip: You can serve this with sliced fresh avocado, atop sandwich bread, or rolled into a warmed tortilla. Older children and other family members may enjoy it with crispy tortillas or pita chips.

Feel-Good Chicken and Wild Rice Soup

SERVES 8

Prep time:
30 minutes

Cook time:
45 minutes

Freezer-Friendly

Healthy Fats

Nut-Free

This recipe is a hug in a bowl, with tender chunks of chicken, flavorful herbed rice, and crispy bacon crumbles all swimming in a rich, creamy broth. The thick consistency of this soup is a great starter for self-feeders because it clings well to spoons, and every bite is full of nutrients. As dietitians, we emphasize that food is the literal fuel for our bodies' growth, healing, and development, and we encourage families to model intuitive eating and listening to their bodies at mealtime, not calorie counting. This recipe makes a generous amount of soup and freezes well for future meals.

4 cups low-sodium chicken broth

2 cups water

1 (4-ounce) box wild rice, rinsed

½ cup diced onion

8 tablespoons (1 stick) unsalted butter

1 cup unbleached all-purpose flour

½ teaspoon sea salt

1 tablespoon chopped fresh rosemary, or 1 teaspoon dried rosemary

½ teaspoon freshly ground black pepper

2 cups half-and-half, or 1 cup heavy cream plus 1 cup whole milk

2 cups shredded cooked chicken

8 slices crispy cooked bacon, crumbled

1. In a large stockpot over medium-high heat, combine the broth, water, wild rice, and onion. Bring the liquid to a low boil, then reduce the heat to medium-low. Cover and simmer about 30 minutes, or until the rice is almost tender but hasn't absorbed all the liquid.
2. Meanwhile, make a roux by melting the butter in a medium saucepan over medium heat. Once the butter has completely melted, quickly whisk in the flour, salt, rosemary, and pepper. It will immediately begin to thicken. Whisk continually until smooth and golden brown, about 2 to 3 minutes.
3. Gradually whisk the half-and-half into the roux and continue to whisk while the mixture thickens and clings to the whisk, about 5 minutes.
4. Transfer the roux into the stockpot and stir to incorporate. Add the shredded chicken and bacon crumbles and stir. Reduce the heat to low and cook, stirring about every 5 minutes, for about 10 minutes, or until the desired thickness is reached.
5. Store in a sealed container in the refrigerator for up to 3 days or freeze for up to 3 months.

Tip: Typically with soups, the slower they're cooked, the better. This allows more time for the flavors to take hold and to cook off excess liquid, giving the soup an extra-creamy texture. This soup can be prepped and then transferred to a slow cooker set on low for slow afternoon cooking, or it can stay on the stovetop over low heat for as long as desired. Soup freezes wonderfully and can always be thinned out with extra water, milk, or broth when reheated.

Black Bean, Corn, and Zucchini Lazy Enchiladas

SERVES 6

Prep time:
15 minutes

Cook time:
35 minutes

Freezer-Friendly

Healthy Fats

Nut-Free

Vegetarian

What's lazy about these enchiladas you ask? No need to fill and roll individual tortillas; simply layer and go. This fool-proof homemade enchilada sauce comes together surprisingly quickly and can also be used to top nachos or burrito bowls.

2 tablespoons olive oil

2 tablespoons unbleached all-purpose flour

1½ cups low-sodium vegetable broth

1 (15-ounce) can crushed tomatoes, no salt added

2 tablespoons tomato paste

1 tablespoon chili powder

1 teaspoon garlic powder

1 teaspoon ground cumin

¼ teaspoon sea salt

1 (15-ounce) can low-sodium black beans, drained and rinsed

1 large zucchini, chopped (about 2 cups)

1 cup corn (fresh or frozen)

3 cups grated sharp cheddar cheese (about 12 ounces), divided

12 (6-inch) corn tortillas

Cilantro, pickled onions, thinly sliced radishes, sliced avocado, and plain whole milk yogurt, for serving

1. Preheat the oven to 350°F.
2. In a small saucepan, heat the oil over medium heat. Whisk in the flour to form a roux. Whisk the roux continually and watch it closely to avoid burning. Cook for about 2 to 3 minutes, or until golden brown.

3. Whisk in the broth, tomatoes, tomato paste, chili powder, garlic powder, cumin, and salt. Bring to a simmer and cook for 2 to 3 minutes, stirring often, then reduce the heat to low and continue simmering the enchilada sauce for 5 minutes more, stirring occasionally, until thickened.

4. In a medium bowl, combine the black beans, zucchini, and corn. Add ¼ cup of enchilada sauce and 1 cup of cheese and stir to mix.

5. Pour ½ cup of enchilada sauce into a 9-by-13-inch baking dish and spread it evenly over the bottom of the pan. Place 4 tortillas over the sauce. Top with 2½ cups of bean filling, 4 more tortillas, ½ cup of sauce, 2½ cups of filling, the remaining 4 tortillas, ½ cup of sauce, and the remaining filling. Top with the remaining sauce and the remaining 2 cups of cheese.

6. Bake for 20 to 25 minutes, or until the cheese has melted and begins to turn golden brown and the edges are bubbly.

7. Store leftovers in the refrigerator for up to 3 days or freeze, either before or after baking, for up to 3 months.

Crispy Tofu Nuggets and Coconut Rice

SERVES 4

Prep time:
20 minutes

Cook time:
20 minutes

Healthy Fats

Vegetarian

While visiting a fruit plantation on the Hawaiian island of Maui, Ellen learned that, despite modern technology, every coconut must be husked by hand. There is no machine that can predict the shape and size of a coconut. Each one is perfectly unique. Since that trip her love for coconut has reached new heights, leading to constant cravings for coconut and endless recipe experiments—which brings us to this crispy coconut tofu with sweet and creamy rice.

For the coconut rice

1 (13½-ounce) can
   full-fat coconut milk
2 cups water
2 cups jasmine rice, rinsed

½ teaspoon sea salt
3 tablespoons unsweetened
   flaked coconut
1 tablespoon coconut oil

For the tofu nuggets

1 (14-ounce) package
   extra-firm tofu
½ cup whole wheat flour
½ teaspoon sea salt
½ teaspoon freshly
   ground black pepper

3 large eggs
1 cup panko bread crumbs
1 cup unsweetened
   shredded coconut
2 to 3 tablespoons coconut
   oil, for frying

1. **To make the coconut rice:** In a medium saucepan, combine the coconut milk and water and bring to a low boil over medium-high heat. Add the rice, salt, unsweetened coconut, and coconut oil. Stir to combine.

2. Bring back to a boil, then reduce the heat to low. Cover and cook for about 10 minutes, or until all the liquid is absorbed. Stir. Remove from the heat and let sit, covered, for about 10 minutes. Uncover and fluff the rice with a fork.

3. Store the rice in a sealed container in the refrigerator for up to 3 days.

4. **To make the tofu nuggets:** Wrap the entire piece of tofu in a clean dishcloth or paper towels and put it on a plate or cutting board. Set a heavy object, like a cast-iron skillet, on top. After about 5 minutes, switch to a dry section of the towel or rewrap the tofu in new paper towels. Set the heavy object on top again. Press the tofu in this way for about 15 minutes total. The towels should be saturated.

5. In the meantime, gather 3 medium bowls. In the first bowl, combine the flour, salt, and pepper. Beat the eggs together in the second bowl. In the third bowl, combine the panko and shredded coconut.

6. Make sure the tofu is thoroughly dry. Cut the tofu into bite-size pieces or about 1-inch chunks. Lay the tofu chunks flat on the towel and give them one more pat to ensure all excess moisture is eliminated.

CONTINUED

7. Set up an assembly line: Coat a piece of tofu in the flour, then thoroughly cover it with egg, and finally, using tongs, generously coat the tofu with the coconut-panko breading. Set the breaded tofu on a clean plate and repeat the process with the remaining "nuggets."

8. Line a large plate with paper towels.

9. In a large cast-iron skillet over medium-high heat, melt 2 tablespoons of coconut oil. Test the oil with a droplet of water; you'll hear a quick sizzle when it's hot enough. Add the coconut nuggets to the oil and cook for about 30 seconds on each side, until they are a beautiful golden brown, adding more oil if necessary. Remove the nuggets from the skillet and set them on the prepared plate to cool.

10. Store in a sealed container in the refrigerator for up to 3 days.

Tip: Drying the tofu is an essential step in this recipe. The more moisture absorbed in the towel, the crispier the tofu cooks up. For older children and adults, these crispy sweet nuggets are delicious paired with sweet 'n' sour or spicy chili dipping sauce.

Cilantro-Lime Chicken Thighs

SERVES 4

Prep time:
5 minutes

Cook time:
40 minutes

Dairy-Free

Freezer-Friendly

Healthy Fats

Iron-Rich

Nut-Free

On the Go

Chicken thighs cook up so flavorful and tender and also feature more iron than white meat. In addition, chicken thighs are one of the more budget-friendly meats in the grocery store. To serve to toddler, cut these into bite-size pieces or shred the meat.

3 tablespoons olive oil

¼ cup minced fresh cilantro

2 cloves garlic, minced

2 tablespoons lime juice

1 teaspoon lime zest

1 teaspoon chili powder

1 teaspoon ground cumin

¼ teaspoon sea salt

1½ pounds skin-on, bone-in chicken thighs

1. Preheat the oven to 425°F. Line a rimmed baking sheet with parchment paper.
2. In a small bowl, whisk together the oil, cilantro, garlic, lime juice, lime zest, chili powder, cumin, and salt.
3. Arrange the chicken thighs on the prepared baking sheet and drizzle with the oil mixture, using your clean hands to ensure the chicken is evenly coated.
4. Roast for 35 to 40 minutes, or until the internal temperature reaches 165°F and the chicken is golden brown.
5. Store leftovers in a sealed container in the refrigerator for up to 3 days or freeze for up to 3 months.

Tip: For even more flavor, put the chicken in a large zip-top bag or sealable container with the cilantro, lime, and olive oil marinade and let it sit in the refrigerator overnight before cooking.

Aunt Marge's Classic Italian Meatballs

SERVES 4 TO 6

Prep time:
10 minutes

Cook time:
25 minutes

Early Introduction

Freezer-Friendly

Healthy Fats

Iron-Rich

Nut-Free

There is something so empowering when someone asks, "Did you make this from scratch?" and you can finally say, "*Yes!*" In some families, cooking together is almost a rite of passage, a mini time warp into someone else's past. Family secrets are shared, emotional bonds are strengthened, and life lessons are learned. If you have a rich heritage like this, don't let it slip by. Talk to your family and cook with them. If you do not have culinary traditions in your family, dare to create some of your own.

2 cups Italian bread crumbs
1 cup minced onion
1 pound ground beef
½ pound ground sausage
½ cup chopped fresh parsley
½ cup freshly grated
   Parmesan cheese

1 tablespoon minced garlic
Sea salt (optional)
Freshly ground black
   pepper (optional)
1 tablespoon olive oil

1. Preheat the oven to 350°F. Line a rimmed baking sheet with parchment paper.
2. In a large mixing bowl, mix together the bread crumbs and onion.
3. Add the ground beef, sausage, parsley, Parmesan, garlic, and salt and pepper (if using).
4. With clean hands, gently blend the mixture until just combined, but make sure all of the ingredients are thoroughly incorporated. Be careful not to overwork the meat.

5. To form a meatball, wet your hands in lukewarm water, then fill ¼-cup measuring cup with meat mixture. Turn the meat out into your hands and roll it into a smooth ball, then set it on a large plate. Repeat until all of the meat mixture has been used (you should have about 18 meatballs).

6. In a large cast-iron skillet, heat the oil over medium-high heat. Lightly brown the meatballs for 2 to 3 minutes, using tongs to turn them and making sure they are evenly browned on all sides. Transfer the meatballs to the prepared baking sheet, setting them about 1 inch apart.

7. Bake for 15 to 20 minutes, or until the meatballs reach an internal temperature of 160°F.

8. Store leftovers in a sealed container in the refrigerator for up to 3 days or freeze in a large container or individual portions for up to 3 months.

Tip: Using these meatballs for a classic Italian pasta? Instead of baking them in the oven, they can be browned, tossed into your favorite simmering spaghetti sauce, and cooked for 15 to 20 minutes or until they reach an internal temperature of 160°F.

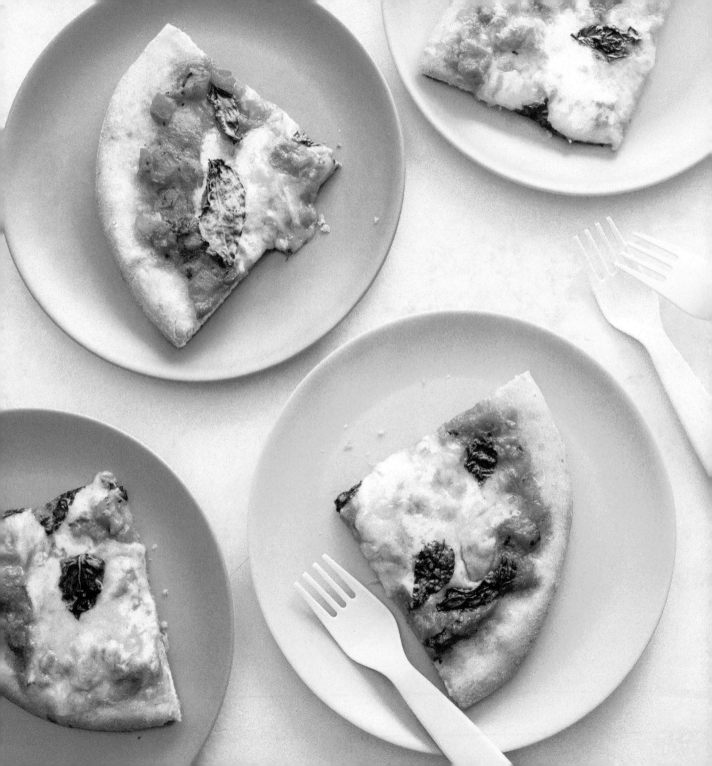

Thin-Crust Margherita Pizza

**MAKES
2 (10-INCH)
THIN-CRUST
PIZZAS**

**Prep time:
30 minutes,
plus 1 hour
30 minutes
to rise**

**Cook time:
15 minutes**

Early Introduction

Freezer-Friendly

Healthy Fats

Nut-Free

Vegetarian

Pizza is an absolute favorite meal for making and eating together as a family. We want to provide a trusted crust recipe for your family to turn to on pizza night. Customize the toppings to your liking and double the recipe to make four 10-inch pizzas.

1 cup warm water (about 110°F)

1 (¼-ounce) packet active dry yeast (about 2¼ teaspoons)

1 teaspoon sugar

1 cup whole wheat flour

1½ cups unbleached all-purpose flour, plus more for dusting

½ teaspoon sea salt

2 tablespoons olive oil, plus more for greasing

1 teaspoon garlic powder

1 (15-ounce) can crushed tomatoes, no salt added

2 (6-ounce) balls fresh mozzarella cheese, sliced into rounds

1 cup torn or roughly chopped fresh basil leaves

1. Preheat the oven to 450°F.
2. In a large mixing bowl, combine the warm water, yeast, and sugar and let them sit for 5 to 10 minutes, or until foamy. If the mixture doesn't get foamy, it means the yeast is no longer fresh and you'll need to start again with another packet.
3. Stir the whole wheat flour, all-purpose flour, and salt into the yeast mixture, bringing it together with your clean hands. Transfer the dough to a lightly floured sheet of parchment paper on a table or countertop. Knead the dough for 2 to 3 minutes, or until it is soft and elastic. If the dough is still sticky, add more all-purpose flour, 1 tablespoon at a time.

CONTINUED

4. Coat the inside of a large, clean bowl with olive oil and cover the dough on all sides in the oil. Put the dough into the bowl, cover it tightly with plastic wrap, and allow the dough to rise until doubled in size, about 1 hour 30 minutes.

5. Divide the dough into 2 equal-size balls and move each one to its own sheet of parchment paper. Using a rolling pin, roll each ball of dough into a large, thin circle about 10 inches in diameter.

6. Transfer each piece of parchment paper with the crust on top to a baking sheet. Drizzle 1 tablespoon of olive oil over each crust, then sprinkle the garlic powder evenly over each crust. Top each pizza with half of the crushed tomatoes, sliced mozzarella, and fresh basil.

7. Bake for 10 to 15 minutes, or until the crust is browned and crispy and the cheese is bubbly and golden.

8. Store leftovers in a sealed container in the refrigerator for up to 3 days. To freeze the dough, wrap it tightly in plastic wrap, place it in a freezer-safe bag, and freeze for up to 3 months. To freeze an unbaked assembled pizza, wrap the pan tightly with plastic wrap and freeze for up to 1 month for best quality.

Tip: Fresh cheeses like the mozzarella in this recipe are much lower in sodium than aged cheeses like Parmesan. Fresh mozzarella also has a soft texture, making it a great choice for babies 6 months and older.

Sunday Roast

**SERVES
4 TO 6**

**Prep time:
15 minutes**

**Cook time:
2 to 3 hours**

Iron-Rich

Nut-Free

We love recipes like this with hands-off cooking, allowing more time with friends and family. Family meals are sacred, and bringing a new baby into the family is the perfect time to reinvent what mealtime can look like in your home. Set your own standards, make your own traditions, and build beautiful memories.

1 (2- to 3-pound) chuck roast
Sea salt
Freshly ground black pepper
2 tablespoons olive oil
1 tablespoon minced garlic
2 cups low-sodium beef broth
5 or 6 celery stalks
1 large onion, sliced

5 or 6 whole carrots
1 tablespoon chopped fresh rosemary, or 1 teaspoon dried rosemary
1 tablespoon fresh thyme leaves, or 1 teaspoon dried thyme

1. Preheat the oven to 275°F.
2. Generously season the roast with salt and pepper on all sides.
3. In a Dutch oven (preferably cast-iron, if you have it), heat the oil and garlic over medium-high heat. When the oil is hot, add the meat and sear it all over, about 2 minutes on each side. Add the broth, celery, onion, carrots, rosemary, and thyme. Cover, transfer to the oven, and cook for about 1 hour per each pound of the roast, or until the meat is tender and falling apart.
4. Store leftovers in a sealed container in the refrigerator for up to 3 days.

Tip: This Sunday roast tastes great atop mashed potatoes; to save time, about halfway through cooking, throw in a couple of potatoes that are roughly cut into chunks.

Tuscan-Inspired Chicken with Spinach and Sun-Dried Tomatoes

SERVES 4 TO 6

Prep time:
10 minutes

Cook time:
30 minutes

Freezer-Friendly

Healthy Fats

This single-skillet dinner is so flavorful and filling. The tender chicken thighs are great for young eaters, and the sauce is packed with healthy calories. This spoon-lickin'-good skillet entree is delicious served over quinoa, couscous, or cauliflower rice.

1 to 1½ pounds boneless, skinless chicken thighs

¼ teaspoon sea salt, plus more for the sauce

⅛ teaspoon freshly ground black pepper, plus more for the sauce

½ teaspoon garlic powder

¼ teaspoon onion powder

1 tablespoon coconut oil

½ cup chopped onion

1 tablespoon minced garlic

1 tablespoon unbleached all-purpose flour

1 cup low-sodium chicken broth

¾ cup full-fat coconut milk

1 teaspoon ground mustard

1 tablespoon fresh parsley, or 1 teaspoon dried parsley

½ tablespoon fresh oregano, or ½ teaspoon dried oregano

⅔ cup chopped sun-dried tomatoes

1½ cups chopped baby spinach

Cooked quinoa, couscous, or rice of choice, for serving

1. Season the chicken thighs with salt, pepper, garlic powder, and onion powder. In a large cast-iron skillet, melt the coconut oil over medium-high heat. Once it is hot, add the chicken thighs and cook for about 5 minutes on each side, or until they are browned and the internal temperature reaches 165°F. Remove the chicken from the skillet and set aside.
2. In the same skillet over medium heat, use the drippings from the chicken to sauté the onion and garlic for 3 to 5 minutes, or until the onions are translucent and beginning to brown.
3. Whisk in the flour to create a roux and cook, whisking continually, for 2 to 3 minutes, until smooth. Whisk in the chicken broth and coconut milk, then add the mustard, parsley, oregano, and salt and pepper to taste. Bring to a low boil and cook on medium-high heat, continuing to whisk, until it starts to thicken, about 5 minutes.
4. Stir in the chopped sun-dried tomatoes and spinach. The sun-dried tomatoes will soak up the juice and begin to soften, and the spinach will immediately begin to wilt. Cook for 3 to 4 minutes, then add the chicken thighs back to the skillet and simmer for another 2 minutes.
5. Serve over quinoa, couscous, or your rice of choice.
6. Store leftovers in a sealed container in the refrigerator for up to 3 days or freeze a large container or individual portions for up to 3 months.

Baby Bolognese with Spaghetti Squash

This is an iron-rich match made in heaven: nutrient-dense beef and vitamin C–rich tomato. We talk about iron a lot because it is the most important nutrient for little eaters. Iron needs are highest for babies between 6 and 12 months, coming in at 11 milligrams per day. Because not much food actually makes it into the mouths of many babies at this age, we aim to make each bite as nutrient packed as possible.

For the Bolognese sauce

1 tablespoon olive oil

2 garlic cloves, minced

1 onion, finely chopped

1 cup grated carrot (about 1 large or 2 medium carrots)

1 pound ground beef

1 (28-ounce) can crushed tomatoes, no salt added

½ cup heavy (whipping) cream

1 teaspoon fresh thyme leaves, or ½ teaspoon dried thyme

For the spaghetti squash

1 spaghetti squash

2 tablespoons unsalted butter

1. **To make the Bolognese sauce:** In a large saucepan or cast-iron skillet, heat the oil over medium heat. Add the garlic and onion and sauté for about 5 minutes, or until softened and fragrant.

2. Add the carrot, cover, and cook, stirring often, for 3 to 5 minutes, or until fork-tender. Add the ground beef and cook, breaking it up into very small pieces as it cooks, until browned, about 7 minutes.

3. Add the crushed tomatoes, cream, and thyme. Cover and simmer for at least 20 minutes, stirring often, until very tender.

4. Allow to cool slightly before serving or storing. Refrigerate leftovers in a sealed container for up to 3 days or freeze for up to 3 months.

5. **To make the spaghetti squash:** While the sauce is cooking, pierce the whole spaghetti squash with a fork and microwave on high for 15 minutes.

6. Remove the squash from the microwave and allow it to cool slightly. Slice it in half, remove the seeds, and use a fork to scrape out the flesh of the squash so that it becomes stringy, like noodles. Transfer to a serving bowl and mix in the butter.

7. Store leftovers in a sealed container in the refrigerator for up to 3 days or freeze for up to 3 months.

Tip: To serve this dish to a baby who is still enjoying purees, scoop some of the flesh from the squash and puree it with water, low-sodium broth, or cream until it reaches a smooth consistency. Serve with Bolognese sauce.

Baked Salmon Fish Sticks

The frozen versions of this classic kid food are convenient, but they often have so many ingredients it makes you wonder how much fish is actually in there. Try out this omega-3-rich homemade version featuring budget-friendly frozen salmon. This recipe works equally well with other firm fish such as cod or tilapia.

1½ pounds frozen skinless salmon, thawed and patted dry
1 egg
2 cups panko bread crumbs
¼ teaspoon sea salt
¼ teaspoon freshly ground black pepper
¼ cup olive oil

1. Preheat the oven to 400°F. Line a rimmed baking sheet with parchment paper.
2. Cut the salmon into 1- to 1½-inch-thick strips.
3. Gather 2 small bowls. In the first bowl, lightly beat the egg. In the second bowl, combine the panko, salt, and pepper.
4. Set up an assembly line: One by one, dip the salmon strips in the egg and then roll them in the bread crumbs, coating the fish evenly and thoroughly. Gently tap off any excess breading and place the fish sticks on the prepared baking sheet.
5. Drizzle the olive oil over the fish sticks and use your clean hands to roll the fish sticks around to ensure all the breading is coated with oil.
6. Bake for 15 to 20 minutes, flipping halfway through, until the fish sticks are lightly browned on all sides.
7. Store leftovers in a sealed container in the refrigerator for up to 3 days or freeze for up to 3 months.

Green Monster Pasta

SERVES 4

Prep time:
15 minutes

Cook time:
15 minutes

Early Introduction

Healthy Fats

Iron-Rich

Quick and Easy

Vegetarian

We know from our experience creating menus for school meal programs that giving something new a fun name can help with acceptance. You can involve little ones by letting them pour their own sauce over a bowl of noodles (don't be discouraged if they try only a little bit at first!).

1 garlic clove
2 cups loosely packed
    fresh basil leaves
4 cups loosely packed
    fresh spinach leaves
½ cup chopped walnuts
    or pecans
½ cup shredded
    Parmesan cheese

½ teaspoon sea salt
½ cup olive oil
¼ cup heavy
    (whipping) cream
2 tablespoons fresh
    lemon juice
1 (16-ounce) box small
    pasta, such as spirals
    or mini shells

1. Fill a large stockpot two-thirds full with water. Bring the water to a boil over high heat.
2. In a blender or food processor, combine the garlic, basil, spinach, nuts, Parmesan, and salt and pulse while slowly streaming in the olive oil, scraping down the sides as needed. When all of the olive oil is incorporated, add the cream and lemon juice and pulse until combined.
3. Cook the pasta according to the package instructions for al dente. Drain and allow it to cool slightly. Place the pasta in a serving bowl, pour the sauce on top, and toss to coat.
4. Leftovers can be stored in a sealed container in the refrigerator for up to 3 days.

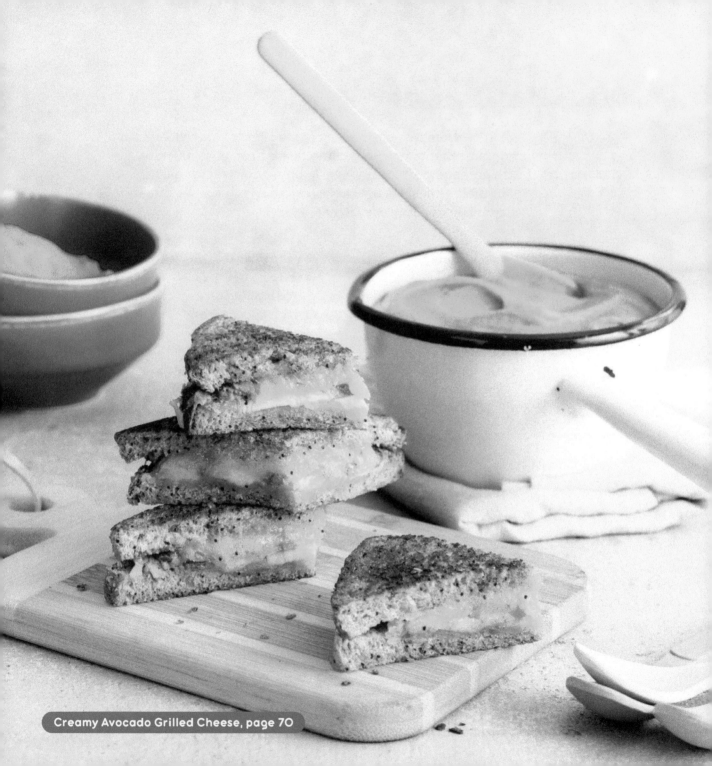

Creamy Avocado Grilled Cheese, page 70

Healthy Meal Builder

Read this chart from left to right to form nutritious food combinations for baby. Each row constitutes one meal.

IRON-RICH FOODS	ESSENTIAL FATS	COLORFUL FRUITS AND VEGGIES	SPICES AND SEASONINGS
Canned salmon, flaked or mashed	Olive oil	Mashed cauliflower	Lemon and garlic
Steamed kale	Scrambled egg	Fresh raspberries	Black pepper
Flaked sardines	Cheese and crackers	Diced kiwi	Cilantro
Lentils	Coconut oil	Thinly sliced sautéed spinach	Turmeric and ginger
Mashed black beans	Mashed avocado	Mashed tomato	Cumin
Mashed chickpeas	Olive oil	Soft pear slices	Cinnamon
Mashed pinto beans	Shredded cheddar cheese	Mashed avocado	Cumin and chili powder
Oatmeal	Almond butter	Strawberries	Nutmeg
Oatmeal	Butter	Applesauce	Cinnamon
Soaked chia seeds	Peanut butter	Banana	Cardamom
Pumpkin puree	Whole milk yogurt	Banana	Cinnamon
Slow-cooked chicken, shredded	Avocado slices	Sliced tomato	Basil

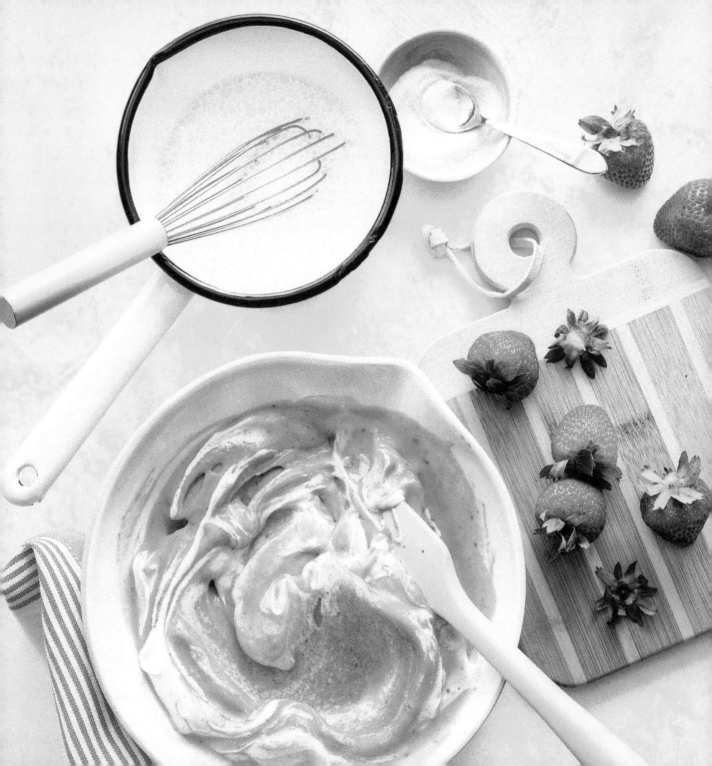

Measurement Conversions

VOLUME EQUIVALENTS (LIQUID)

US Standard	US Standard (ounces)	Metric (approximate)
2 tablespoons	1 fl. oz.	30 mL
¼ cup	2 fl. oz.	60 mL
½ cup	4 fl. oz.	120 mL
1 cup	8 fl. oz.	240 mL
1½ cups	12 fl. oz.	355 mL
2 cups or 1 pint	16 fl. oz.	475 mL
4 cups or 1 quart	32 fl. oz.	1 L
1 gallon	128 fl. oz.	4 L

OVEN TEMPERATURES

Fahrenheit	Celsius (approximate)
250°F	120°C
300°F	150°C
325°F	165°C
350°F	180°C
375°F	190°C
400°F	200°C
425°F	220°C
450°F	230°C

VOLUME EQUIVALENTS (DRY)

US Standard	Metric (approximate)
⅛ teaspoon	0.5 mL
¼ teaspoon	1 mL
½ teaspoon	2 mL
¾ teaspoon	4 mL
1 teaspoon	5 mL
1 tablespoon	15 mL
¼ cup	59 mL
⅓ cup	79 mL
½ cup	118 mL
⅔ cup	156 mL
¾ cup	177 mL
1 cup	235 mL
2 cups or 1 pint	475 mL
3 cups	700 mL
4 cups or 1 quart	1 L

WEIGHT EQUIVALENTS

US Standard	Metric (approximate)
½ ounce	15 g
1 ounce	30 g
2 ounces	60 g
4 ounces	115 g
8 ounces	225 g
12 ounces	340 g
16 ounces or 1 pound	455 g

Resources

Division of Responsibility in Feeding, EllynSatterInstitute.org: Much more information from the founder of the Division of Responsibility, Ellyn Satter, on raising happy, healthy eaters and reducing picky eating behaviors.

How to Start an Herb Garden, TastefulGarden.com/Herb -Gardening-for-Beginners-d19.htm: Growing your own herbs is an inexpensive and healthy way to add flavor variety for your little one.

Intuitive Eating, EvelynTribole.com/resources/intuitive-eating -resources: Authoring her first book on Intuitive Eating in 1995, Evelyn Tribole, MS, RDN, CEDRD-S, leads the way in Intuitive Education for adults.

Local Harvest, LocalHarvest.org: An easy-to-use directory for finding local produce, meat, dairy, and CSA programs based on your zip code. The site also provides links to each farm's website for detailed information about how the produce or animals are raised.

Mama Knows Nutrition, @mamaknows_nutrition, and **Kids Eat in Color, @kids.eat.in.color:** Trustworthy Instagram accounts featuring reliable, approachable information on feeding babies and toddlers.

Square One Wellness, SquareOneWellness.net, and **Morton's Grove, MortonsGrove.com:** Stuck on what foods to offer next? Check out our blogs and workshops (online and in person) for many more first-food ideas to offer your baby and toddler, from the first few months through the first few years.

References

Abrams, Elissa, and Allan Becker. "Food Introduction and Allergy Prevention in Infants." *Canadian Medical Association Journal* 187, no. 17 (November 17, 2015): 1297–1301. doi: 10.1503/cmaj.150364.

American Academy of Pediatrics. "Infant Food and Feeding." AAP.org/en-us/advocacy-and-policy/aap-health-initiatives/HALF-Implementation-Guide/Age-Specific-Content/Pages/Infant-Food-and-Feeding.aspx.

Bennet, William, Kristin Hendrix, Rachel Thompson, Stephen Downs, and Aaron Carroll. "Early Cow's Milk Introduction Is Associated with Failed Personal-Social Milestones after One Year of Age." *European Journal of Pediatrics* 173, no. 7 (July 2014): 887–92. doi: 10.1007/s00431-014-2265-y.

Centers for Disease Control and Prevention (CDC). "Antibiotic/Antimicrobial Resistance (AR/AMR): Food and Food Animals." Updated February 10, 2020. CDC.gov/drugresistance/food.html.

De Cosmi, Valentina, Silvia Scaglioni, and Carlo Agostoni. "Early Taste Experiences and Later Food Choices." *Nutrients* 9, no. 2 (February 2017): 107. doi: 10.3390/nu9020107.

Eat Right Pro (Academy of Nutrition and Dietetics). "The Right Time to Start Infants on Solid Foods: New Study in Journal of the Academy of Nutrition and Dietetics." January 4, 2018. EatRightPro.org/media/press-releases/new-in-food-nutrition-and-health/when-is-the-right-time-to-start-infants-on-solid-foods.

Harnack, Lisa, Mary Cogswell, James Shikany, Christopher Gardner, Cathleen Gillespie, Catherine Loria, et al. "Sources of Sodium in US Adults from 3 Geographic Regions." *Circulation* 135, no. 19 (May 9, 2017): 1775–83. doi: 10.1161/CIRCULATIONAHA.116.024446.

HealthyChildren.org (American Academy of Pediatrics). "Where We Stand: Fruit Juice." Updated May 19, 2017. HealthyChildren.org/English/healthy-living/nutrition/Pages/Where-We-Stand-Fruit-Juice.aspx.

Iweala, Onyinye, Shaliesh K. Choudhary, and Scott P. Commins. "Food Allergy." *Current Gastroenterology Reports* 20, no. 5 (April 5, 2018): 17. doi: 10.1007/s11894-018-0624-y.

Johns Hopkins Medicine. "Food Allergies in Children." HopkinsMedicine.org/health/conditions-and-diseases/food-allergies-in-children.

Liu, Jianghong. "Eating Fish Linked to Better Sleep and Higher IQ in Children." National Institute of Environmental Health Sciences. Updated February 7, 2018. niehs.nih.gov/research/supported/sep/2018/eating-fish/index.cfm.

Park View Pediatrics. "Food Allergies and Your Child." 2007. ParkViewPediatricsCO.com/Education/Nutrition/Food-Allergies-and-Your-Child.

Petts, Jennifer. "Can I Prevent My Baby from Getting Food Allergies?" The Iowa Clinic. February 6, 2020. IowaClinic.com/allergy/can-food-allergies-be-prevented-in-kids.

Sicherer, Scott. "New Guidelines Detail Use of 'Infant-Safe' Peanut to Prevent Allergy." *AAP News*, January 5, 2017. AAPPublications.org/news/2017/01/05/PeanutAllergy010517.

Togias, Alkis, Susan F. Cooper, Maria L. Acebal, Amal Assa'ad, James R. Baker, Lisa A. Beck, et al. "Addendum Guidelines for the Prevention of Peanut Allergy in the United States: Report of the National Institute of Allergy and Infectious Diseases—Sponsored Expert Panel." *World Allergy Organization Journal* 10, no.1 (January 2017): 1. doi: 10.1186/s40413-016-0137-9.

Trasande, Leonardo, Rachel M. Shaffer, and Sheela Sathyanarayana. "Food Additives and Child Health." *Pediatrics* 142 (2): e20181408. doi: 10.1542/peds.2018-1408.

US Food and Drug Administration. "Steroid Hormone Implants Used for Growth in Food-Producing Animals." Updated April 20, 2020. FDA.gov/animal-veterinary/product-safety-information/steroid-hormone-implants-used-growth-food-producing-animals.

World Health Organization. "Food, Genetically Modified." WHO.int/health-topics/food-genetically-modified/#tab=tab_1.

World Health Organization. "Infant and Young Child Feeding." Updated April 1, 2020. WHO.int/news-room/fact-sheets/detail/infant-and-young-child-feeding.

Index

Acknowledgments

Laura

Thank you to my family, especially to both Mimis, for helping me accomplish this book. To Ruthie and Bobby, my adventurous eaters. To all of the dietitians out there for paving the way for us while sharing nutrition advice as reliable as it is awesome. And to my great friend and coauthor, Ellen, for driving to my house to test recipes until we didn't have a clean dish left.

Ellen

This writing process is one I'll never forget, as years' worth of life events transpired over mere weeks. From grocery shopping during a global pandemic to testing recipes without a functioning kitchen, announcing a new addition to the family, and consequently editing content from a hospital bed, thank you to my family and friends for always cheering me on through seemingly impossible tasks. To my husband, Steve, and daughter, Ruth, the two best friends anyone could have, I love you. To my coauthor, Laura, you are the backbone of this project. Let's keep saying yes together!

About the Authors

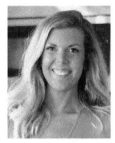

Laura Morton, **MS**, **RDN**, **LD**, is a registered dietitian and mom to two adventurous toddlers. She shares budget-friendly whole food recipes and her journey to peaceful mealtimes on her blog, Morton's Grove. Laura believes the goal with feeding, as in other areas of parenting, is to cultivate a healthy relationship with food that lasts a lifetime. She shares this approach when counseling families with babies and toddlers. Laura and her family live in a 100-year-old farmhouse way out in the country, where you will almost always find them running around barefoot.

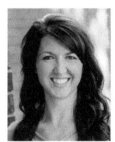

Ellen Gipson, **MA**, **RDN**, **LD**, is a registered dietitian, mom, and self-identified super taster. From a dietetics career in school nutrition to her current pursuit of infant and family nutrition education and counseling with her company, Square One Wellness, Ellen champions the philosophy that food isn't nutritious unless eaten, and early (and continual) exposure is essential in establishing healthy eating habits. Her first cookbook, *BLW Baby Food Cookbook*, has inspired parents and caregivers across the country to embark upon their own food adventures. She resides in Cape Girardeau, Missouri, with her husband, Steve, three-year-old daughter, Ruth, and the most prideful cat, Mr. Darcy.

CPSIA information can be obtained
at www.ICGtesting.com
Printed in the USA
BVHW020852051120
592600BV00016B/442